# ADHD Life Is Beautiful

## A True Story

### NICO J. GENES

ADHD: Life Is Beautiful
A True Story
by NICO J. GENES

Published by Nico J. Genes, 2019
Copyright © 2019 Nico J. Genes
All rights reserved.
First edition

ISBN: 9781093629477
Edited by Stephanie Tillman

This is a work of nonfiction based on a true story. Some places, names, and identifying details have been changed in order to maintain the anonymity of other.

This book has been published with all reasonable efforts taken to make the material error-free. No part of this book shall be used or otherwise reproduced in any manner whatsoever without written permission from the author, except in the case of brief quotations embodied in critical articles and reviews.

Nico J. Genes asserts the moral right to be identified as the author of this work.

Enjoy your reading.

## Dedication

*Life is beautiful, dear boy, especially since I met you and your mother.*
*You both enriched my life at so many levels, and I don't think I will ever be able to thank you enough.*
*The words that would capture the depth of my feelings haven't been invented yet.*

# Contents

|    | Prologue | vii |
|----|----------|-----|
| 1  | A Perfect Day | 1 |
| 2  | Surprise, Surprise | 11 |
| 3  | Who Was She? | 18 |
| 4  | My Sweet, Angry Friend | 24 |
| 5  | Nickelodeon Rules | 33 |
| 6  | Are There Any Pigs in Italy? | 43 |
| 7  | Gardaland | 53 |
| 8  | Who Invented School? | 61 |
| 9  | I Hate Myself | 72 |
| 10 | Friends for Life | 79 |
| 11 | Flowers Have Lives Too | 87 |
| 12 | Is Anything More Important Than Your Health? | 93 |
| 13 | New Beginnings | 101 |
| 14 | ADHD or Bad Behavior? | 111 |
| 15 | What Is ADHD? | 119 |
| 16 | What Is Normal? | 131 |
| 17 | The Moment of Truth | 139 |

| | | |
|---|---|---|
| 18 | Second Chances | 146 |
| 19 | True Friendship Never Dies | 158 |
| 20 | Peter | 171 |
| 21 | Eliza | 182 |
| | Afterword - Life Is Beautiful | 191 |
| | Other Titles by This Author | 195 |
| | About the Author | 198 |

## Prologue

"Did you write something for our literature book?" Peter, my friend's son, asked me one day.

"What do you mean?" I answered, intrigued.

"The other day, my teacher was telling us about an author who had written 'Life is beautiful'. I know it was you," he said in a serious, determined tone.

I laughed. "No, it wasn't me, but there are many people that think like me."

"I'm sure it was you! You are the only one I know who's always saying, 'Life is beautiful'."

"No, there are none of my words in your schoolbook," I said, still amused by his way of thinking.

"Admit it. It was you!" he insisted.

In his little head—he was seven at the time—I was the only person who could have said that. I couldn't take the credit for it, even if it felt like he needed this confirmation quite badly. The whole discussion, his thrilled voice, and his way of thinking made me grin.

"Nico, please admit it," said Eliza, his mother. "He won't let it go until you do."

I knew this boy well. I also knew he wouldn't give in easily. Still, I didn't want to give him wrong information or take the credit for something that wasn't mine.

\*\*\*

I didn't write it in his schoolbook, but I'm writing it in mine. Why?

Life itself tricks us, plays us, misleads us, and even paints one man as a good guy when he may as well be a bad one. Good or bad? Or maybe neither. Maybe life is playing the role it should: forever taking us on a journey where it makes it impossible for us to predict what will happen next.

It makes it difficult to realize, at first sight, what kind of person we are coming in contact with. But maybe that is the way it should be. Knowing and being able to predict everything would make life lose its charm. They say that without sadness, we wouldn't be able to know happiness.

Opposites. Pluses and minuses. Attraction. Rejection. They all have their role.

It is because of the bad people I've met in my life that I became capable of distinguishing who is among the good ones. It is because of simple but meaningful gestures or words or even being silent at the right time that makes us appreciate one good person more than others.

What one appreciates in other is very subjective — something that one person loves may be disliked by others. The best thing about someone could be perceived as the worst by different people. Isn't it ironic? This is how the world is, and we could not and should not do anything about it.

What should be valid and necessary for all of us is to have tolerance, to try to understand, or to just accept. We don't have to like everyone. We should not expect everyone to like us. What we can do is to try to refrain from judgment. Do we see flaws? Maybe they are insignificant. If not, we don't have to have a close relationship with that person.

Do we feel that a specific person drags us down? If there is no sign of possible improvement, then why should we stick around? Do we see qualities? Then we should base our relationships on those factors.

Life is precious; good friends are not numerous, but their actions are significant. Cherish them. Feel grateful for them. Show them that you appreciate them. And do all this as often as possible. Be grateful for the bad ones too, as they helped you see the good ones for who they were. I am grateful for any friend that has come into my life and proved to be in the bad category, because it helped me to recognize and appreciate the good ones.

Eliza and Peter have many flaws, and they require patience and lots of tolerance. But they have many positives qualities, and so, I am grateful for having them in my life.

\*\*\*

"Did you write this?" Peter will ask me one day.

"Yes, I did," I will be able to answer truthfully.

"Why did you do that?" he may ask.

"Because of you and your mother, my best friends forever," I will answer in the blink of an eye. "And because now I know, my life wouldn't be as beautiful if you weren't a part of it," I would add.

"Cool," he might say, seeming proud and shy at the same time.

# 1
# A Perfect Day

It was more than five years ago, but I remember everything so clearly as if it happened yesterday. I was facing a stressful period in my life, and I was using every opportunity to relax, recharge my batteries, and improve my overall physical condition and state of mind. One of the most beneficial ways for me to do this was to visit the seaside. So, I did, more than once. I would go as often as I could. It was only a four-hour drive, so I could easily go there for the weekend.

All I needed was to purchase a bus ticket and pack a small bag. I didn't do anything special. I mainly enjoyed the closeness of the sea and taking a short break from the city. It was just what the mind and body needed: being able to relax and do nothing. No deadlines, no requests, no urgent meetings, no emails, no reports, no phone calls.

It was "me time." Sometimes, I was by myself, but I didn't spend the entire time in solitude. Now and then, I was in contact with a small number of people I knew. There were not many of these, and I did not know them very well. This was fine with me. I could easily go there and spend the time by myself. Still, meeting two certain people over there changed my perspective. "Perspective of what?" you might ask. Of life itself and what really matters.

\*\*\*

Let's take it from the beginning of this special story about an important period of my life.

First, I was introduced to Eliza.

Surprisingly, she became a really good friend within a very short time. She was different than others. I could say that. She was not different in terms of appearance, though. Her slim, athletic body; short, messy, platinum-blonde, pixie-cut hair, and big blue eyes were indeed striking, but there was more to her that would grab people's attention. It was her personality that made her stand out.

Eliza seemed to be a non-complicated person who was always ready to jump when needed. On the other hand, she was shy, always smiling, a bit too much, and strange at times. It was a good strange, though.

At first, I didn't understand her constant grin. "What is so funny?" I kept asking. She never had an answer, but she would either smile even more or become serious when I was too persistent with my question.

*'Weird,'* I told myself. I would later learn the reason behind the smile. It didn't take long to notice her gentle personality, kind heart, and everything good in her. The kind attributes of this friend made me quickly overlook any strange behaviors. They were irrelevant.

No one is perfect, right? Are you? I know I'm not.

\*\*\*

Eliza was a social worker who loved her job. She wasn't much of a talker at first, so personal information was revealed slowly, like water dropping from a broken pipe: *drip, drip, drip.*

She was a good listener, though. I like to talk. The perfect combination, it seemed. Despite the fact that she didn't have any experience with my field of work, it felt refreshing to talk through job-related issues with her. Maybe it was exactly because of this that I found her company soothing. I don't know. Looking back, I can find so many reasons why it was good that we'd met, but I can easily remember moments that weren't quite so good. But we got through those moments, and we survived with our friendship intact. I am glad I let her enter my life and am so grateful that she allowed me into hers.

Soon after we met, I was already a regular visitor to the city she lived in. She used a large portion of her precious free time to show me around. She felt the need to protect me and to be my tour guide at the same time. During these days, I didn't speak her language too well, but with the help of the English language, we overcame those barriers. Eliza considered her own English to be very poor, and each time she'd say something in English, her face would turn red. Her perfectly white skin was suddenly blushing. She was cute, though, when she looked embarrassed. Well, at least to me, because, to her, it was a serious issue.

I couldn't believe that someone with her physique and other qualities could have such a low self-esteem. I kept my thoughts to myself at the beginning. I didn't know her that well yet, so I thought I'd better be quiet rather than say something that could be misunderstood. I'm glad I refrained from making comments that may have sounded negative. I know now that she would have taken any comment as a personal criticism.

Despite her mysterious side, Eliza was easygoing, and I felt relaxed in her company. I could be myself the entire time. I could make any suggestions about what we could do together. She was always up for it. She was always not judgmental, unlike other people I knew, and she never pointed out any differences between us. She accepted my needs and choices. I tried to accept hers.

She didn't even make any comments about me being picky about food. It's not a big thing, you might say, but try listening every day over and over again about remarks people say regarding my choice of food, and then you will understand. She was like a breath of fresh air. Someone pleasant to spend time with. Whatever I did or said, she had only nice things to say back or she kept quiet. I did the same.

***

One afternoon, a couple of months after we met, we sat quietly on a pebble beach, facing the beautiful blue sea. It was still winter, but it felt like a lovely spring day. The sun was high in the clear, azure sky. I could feel the rays pleasantly warming my face and body. The sound of the waves crashing onto the shore was relaxing. The wind was blowing gently through my long red hair. Eliza was looking at the expanse of water, lost in her thoughts while I collected stones of different shapes and colors, trying to think about nothing.

"Look at this one," I said, thrilled each time I found another stone, always nicer than the previous one. She would slowly turn her head and would only rarely make a comment.

"This is so silly," she said out of the blue, after many minutes of silence. She wasn't being offensive.

"What is silly?"

"Look at you. You are old enough to have your own children. You are beautiful, smart, successful, and you could have anything you want in life. I'm sure you have many friends that enjoy being in your company. Instead, you are here with me, a nobody, on a pebble beach, and you are collecting stones. You are enjoying them like they are made of gold or some other precious material."

I think this was the longest sentence I'd ever heard from her. She wasn't being sarcastic. She was just describing and pondering exactly what she could see. I couldn't, however, exactly figure out what her stance on all this was.

"You are not a nobody; don't talk like that. I'm really enjoying this, and it relaxes me. To me, these pebbles are precious. They are probably the same as gold is for others," I answered, with a clear expression on my face, enjoying the pleasant, soft breeze that was playing with my hair. It was the truth. I was starting to appreciate things differently during recent years. If I'd met her a few years earlier, I would have probably asked her to go shopping, go for a drink, or to be pampered at a spa. The pebbles, the sea, the salty wind, the sun, and my strange friend were the exact ingredients needed for a perfect day.

We became quiet again. I started singing to myself my own version of the song "Perfect Day" by Lou Reed:

"Just a perfect day
Problems all left alone

Weekenders on our own
It's such fun
Just a perfect day
You made me forget myself…"

The wind blew softly like a melody of joy laying itself all over me, keeping me warm. I let the feeling linger upon me while my hands and eyes still searched for special stones. My singing was interrupted by Eliza's words.

"Don't take me wrong. I love this about you," she said with a calm smile.

"What exactly?" I asked, confused.

"You get happy over little things." I was surprised to hear her noticing this, as earlier, her comment made me feel like she felt the opposite way. Now she seemed to understand. Who knows what was going on in her head? All I know is that she kept smiling and making fun of me each time I got excited for something as insignificant as a seagull flying or the sight of a clear blue sky.

"Why do you laugh then, if you love this about me?" I reacted again to her mixed signals.

"I don't know. This is the way I am," she answered after a short pause.

"What do you mean you don't know? I always know the reason I'm smiling," the rational me replied back.

"Oh, forget it," she brushed me off, making it clear that she had no desire to continue the conversation. The patient Eliza had transformed into a short-tempered, I-don't-want-to-explain person.

\*\*\*

What were we to each other? We were different on so many levels. We lived in different countries. We had different educations. I was ten years older than her, with a more rational look at life. She was still very young.

She was a dreamer and a believer in that everything is possible. She insisted that it is never too late. She believed she could move boulders if she so desired. She enjoyed running, swimming, and riding her bicycle. Eliza was an adrenaline junkie.

I was the opposite. I enjoyed long walks, massages, collecting stones, and admiring roses. Eliza was an adrenaline junkie. I was the opposite. She never had the patience to watch a movie all the way through and barely managed to finish a book. I enjoyed movie marathons and loved reading.

We had different views on so many things. We were different on so many levels and yet so similar on the things that mattered. We were both simple people who believed in the beauty of the world and in the existence of a fair, kindhearted human race. We both had only good intentions and would never be able to hurt anyone on purpose. I think we both managed to see this in each other.

Later on, I would also find out that it was our differences that made our friendship stronger. *Yin and Yang*. We were so different, yet so much alike. Strong, yet so sensitive. Powerful, yet so fragile.

The bottom line was that Eliza was my special friend. With all her weirdness, I thought I still accepted her fully, just the way she was. Boy, was I wrong.

It took me a long time to realize why she was enjoying my company while speaking so little about herself. It was mainly because, unlike all her other friends and relatives, I never criticized her. I always showed her respect. I was calming her down by being patient. I was making her laugh with my many silly ways.

\*\*\*

Back to that afternoon on the beach.

"I have a son," she said suddenly.

"Really? I don't believe you."

"Why not?" she said surprised.

"Because you are too young to be a mother and because you would have mentioned it before."

"Well…" she paused and looked down for a while "…didn't you realize already that I'm different from everyone else you know? There is no logic with me." She almost whispered the last words, and I wasn't sure what exactly she was getting at when she said "different." She did seem different to me, but I wanted to know her definition of it.

"When do I get to meet him?" I asked, instead of saying my thoughts out loud. I was still confused. I knew nothing about her family, but I decided to let her talk about them on her own terms.

"Maybe next time you come here," she answered.

"Great. I need to come as soon as possible, as I would love to meet him." I loved children, so I couldn't wait to meet her baby boy.

"It's a deal," she said, smiling, and I sensed that her happiness was genuine. So, my friend has a child. What other surprises will I discover about her?

Then we fell silent again. This was often how we spent our time together. Sometimes we would talk. Actually, I was often the one doing most of the talking. Other times, we would just stay quiet. It rarely felt awkward, though.

"I could live here," I said, interrupting Eliza's reflective state.

"You should," she said immediately.

"I can't. My job and the rest of my life are elsewhere." Still, I took some time to consider what I'd just said. I loved the place I call home, but it felt so good to be close to the sea whenever I had the chance. Would that feeling stay if I didn't have the feeling that I was on a holiday? I didn't know the answer.

"But you feel so good here. I can feel it."

"That is true, but unfortunately, this is life. I have obligations and commitments at home. I can't just pick things up and go," I said, clearly disappointed.

"You are not aware that you are creating barriers in your head." She spoke these words like she'd known me forever. I was aware that I'm always in control of things. I'm the responsible person. Always the reliable one. As a daughter, sister, cousin, employee, partner or friend, I was always doing my best to meet all the expectations of others. Rarely did I think about things I want for myself. Actually, it was only recently with my short visits to Eliza's home city that I first did something just for myself.

"Maybe you're right. But really, my life is there. This, here, is my 'me time.'"

"Does this mean you may stop coming here?" she asked with a bit of concern on her face.

"No. I will come here every time I get the chance. It isn't that far, and I always go back feeling full of peace and totally relaxed."

She seemed pleased with my answer. Her face relaxed. I wasn't sure how often I could come and for how long. I knew I wanted to, so I wasn't lying.

I breathed in some more sea air, feeling how my lungs embraced it, sending its salted, relaxing signals throughout my body. It felt good. It was unbelievable how my "me time" felt unaltered by her presence. Or maybe it was because of her that I could have this comfortable feeling.

I breathed deeply again and thought, *'Life is beautiful.'*

"We have to go; I'm late," Eliza almost yelled after checking the time. The serenity of the moment was broken in only a second. She hurried to her feet.

"Now?"

"Yes, now. I will have to leave you alone for a while. Will you be okay?"

In a very clumsy way, she collected all the little stones that I'd picked up. I was just beginning to realize that we needed to move. She put some stones in her bag, others in her pockets, while many of them fell on the ground.

"Of course." I wasn't sure she even cared for my answer.

I was out of my comfort zone suddenly. "Where are you going?"

No answer. She was walking quickly, and I barely managed to keep up with her, not bothering with the stones left behind. There will be some more next time. I was glad I wasn't carrying them.

# 2
## Surprise, Surprise

We reached the parking lot, and I was barely sitting down when the car took off. She didn't appear to want to talk. I didn't say anything. At one point, she stopped the car next to a coffee place and told me to go sit and enjoy a coffee while she had something urgent to do.

"When are you coming back?"

Even if she had answered, I never got to hear it, as she drove off Speedy Gonzales-style. The wheels screeched like a racecar. 'Weird,' I told myself again. Still, it didn't bother me. I was going to enjoy my coffee in silence, and that suited me. After all, I didn't even have to sit and wait for her, as I could easily find my way back to my accommodations. My Zen time could continue.

I took out my book and decided to immerse myself in its story while avoiding the temptation to check for work emails. The busy season hadn't started yet, so the place was quiet. The coffee tasted good, and the music in the background was relaxing. The story was interesting. Just when the main character finally discovered she was actually in love with her best friend and confessed, my phone rang.

"Did you drink your coffee? I'm outside. Come on!"

"I'm just—"

She hung up without waiting for my answer. Okay, now it was definitely weird. Still, I stood up, left the money for the coffee on the table, and hurried outside. I saw her car parked very close, and when I approached it, I noticed someone sitting in the back seat.

The moment I opened the door, I was introduced to Peter. I looked at him and his small head covered in curly blond hair. He made me forget about all the recent weird moments.

"Hello," I said to him.

He said nothing.

"What do you say?" Eliza scolded her son.

"Hello," he answered nervously, almost not looking at me.

It didn't bother me, though. "What is your name?" I asked.

"Peter." His voice was a little louder this time.

"Nice to meet you, Peter. My name is Nico." I stretched my hand over the car seat, and he barely touched it. I know some kids will accept me immediately; others need a bit of time. I was still in awe that I'd met him so soon. I found out about his existence only an hour ago, but she'd told me that this would happen on a future visit. I was so happy, in fact, that I totally ignored the weird feeling from earlier.

"How old are you?"

"I'm six," he said proudly.

Once we were back on the road, Eliza explained that she had to take him to a birthday party and that he'd been excited about it all morning. She'd forgotten to check the time. That was the reason for her being in such a hurry. She explained that this didn't happen very often. He was not invited to many parties, so she would never forgive herself if her poor time-keeping caused him to miss it. I found this to be really sad.

In the backseat, he was playing a game on his mother's phone, and it was clear that he was not listening to our conversation, especially because the loud noises of the game would not have allowed him to, even if he had wanted to.

"Why is that? I'm sure he has lots of little friends celebrating their birthdays."

"If you ask him, he will say that everyone is his friend. Unfortunately, not all their parents like Peter, so he often doesn't get invited."

"He seems so sweet. I can't believe anyone would dislike him."

"He is my love. To me, he is the best thing that has ever happened in my life. To others, he often seems just a hyperactive boy with no manners." She was not looking at me while saying these last words, but I could see her face was trying to mask her sadness.

"All children are hyperactive, if you ask me. What manners do they expect from a six-year-old child? Maybe some people expect too much." I didn't have kids of my own, but I felt strongly about this. Eliza didn't comment. I didn't know many things about her, but I knew already that she needed time to open up. If I had one thing, it was patience.

She told me that she'd decided to introduce me to Peter only when she felt that she could fully trust me and was sure I was going to be present in their life on a longer-term basis. But there was something in that moment on the beach that convinced her to do it straight away.

"Peter can be very quick in getting attached to people, so I don't want to make him suffer when they are gone," she explained.

I could understand that and knew she wanted only what was best for her son.

"What are you eating?" I asked Peter in an attempt to make some conversation with him when I noticed he had stopped playing the game.

I was admiring his sweet, big, blue eyes with long eyelashes and curly blonde hair. He looked very much like his mother, but at the age of six, he still had some baby-like features. Just like Eliza, he was almost always moving. He was sometimes quiet and still, and then be exploding with impatience to reach the destination or excitement or nervousness over achieving the next level in his game. He would then become quiet again, looking dazed at something he'd see through the car window. He did all this within a span of twenty minutes.

"Chocolate cream," he answered with a sparkle in his eyes, once he finally considered my earlier question. I looked at his little hands and saw something that looked like two halves of a *Kinder* chocolate egg.

"Can I have some?" I asked with a teasing tone, as I knew that such a small quantity could barely keep his sweet tooth satisfied.

"Yes," he answered immediately.

The moment he handed me one half of his snack, he gained my heart. I couldn't hide the surprise when I saw his little hand passing me the chocolate while I could see only satisfaction on his face, rather than resentment or greed. Such a small gesture could say so much about a person, especially with him being a small child. Maybe I was exaggerating with my enthusiasm, but my feelings were honest. In time, my first impression would be confirmed. I feel my heart melting for the love of this sweet boy each time I think of him.

And this is how I met my two best friends, Eliza and Peter. From that moment onward, I've grown very fond of them. My life reached new dimensions.

\*\*\*

Days, weeks, and months were passing, and visits to my friends' town became a regular thing. Same with spending time with Eliza. On several occasions, I got to see Peter too.

Eliza showed me all the little-known and unknown places in and around her city, and I savored everything with great pleasure. Sometimes we talked about our daily lives, and other times, about life in general. Often, we didn't talk at all. Silence wasn't a bother but was a welcome presence during our moments together. From the moment I reached my getaway destination until the moment I returned home, I was in another world, one that added new meaning to my existence.

With her, I was different than with any of my other friends. I started to enjoy our moments of quietness. Who would have thought I would come to enjoy and feel comfortable with being silent with someone? She helped me realize this without even knowing it.

The other good thing is that even when not talking, I thought about my life, the other life — the one thought I had every time I came back from the seaside. The new "me" was slowly forming there, and those changes gradually transferred to my daily life. Would they have happened even without spending time with my new friends? I don't know.

What I do know is that I was a person feeling and acting differently in my two worlds: the one I had in my own country, with my concerns of material existence, my job, my friends, family, my colleagues, my normal routine; and the other one, with my two new friends, the sea, nature, silence, and attempts at doing or thinking of nothing. Well, almost nothing.

One world asked for and offered notions of a secure, responsible, result-oriented, and, all in all, ordinary life, thoughts, and feelings. The other had no order, no rules, no expectations, no "must do" activities, and yet, it was demanding at times. It was a mix of diverse experiences and feelings.

I found myself smiling, enjoying, and, most importantly, growing more as a person in the latter one. My education, career achievements, connections — none of that was important here. Nothing mattered, except for being a good human being. Why did I feel I belonged to this world more than my original one?

Was it because I was going on mini-vacations, hence the relaxation and enjoyment?

Was it because the closeness of the sea air and nature suited me better?

Was it because I had no deadlines, no obligations, no pressure, and no programs to respect?

Was it because I was free to do what I wanted, whenever I wanted?

Was it because I was taking time to be on my own with my own thoughts and digest them for as long as I needed?

Who was I really? Why did I need such an unusual companionship to start questioning myself more? Or it was a pure coincidence? Have I reached that moment in life when priorities and views change?

Was it then the moment to become more concerned about the purpose of my life? To feel that I had many friends, but only a few were actually the right ones? To decide to make space in life, space for what mattered? How could I become friends with two people so different from me or any of my friends and still feel extremely content, happy, appreciated, and wanted?

The more I asked myself these and similar questions, the closer I got to an answer. It was because of the above and especially due to them, my friends. So different and yet so alike when it came to things that matter. The more I got to know them, the more I discovered how special they were.

# 3
# Who Was She?

Summer came. Spending time at the seaside during the hot days seems to be an appreciated thing, and a common practice, worldwide. In the past, that wasn't for me. I considered myself more of a mountain person. Now, I was using all my free time to be at the seaside. There, I had all I needed to relax and charge my batteries. I also wanted to enjoy more of the beneficial company of my mysterious friend. Always listening, rarely revealing personal stuff. I knew already that she had a low self-esteem, not only from her remarks, not always because she was unable to accept compliments, but because she too often avoided looking me into my eyes. Eye contact is important. It is a sign of self-confidence, trust, honesty, and respect. Did she feel she couldn't confide in me yet?

In time, her trust was building up. Eliza started revealing more. I didn't put any pressure on. It was rare for me to ask. The personal information from "the pipe" was only occasionally going *drip, drip, drip* for me, but it was now happening more often and even pouring more at a time. It wasn't unpleasant like real water floods, as the drips had long waits between them. Sometimes, I couldn't stop from her talking. Not that I tried much, as I was curious to know everything about her. I was the listener in these moments.

## ADHD: LIFE IS BEAUTIFUL

As a child, Eliza was really shy, especially at home with her family. She was always craving more attention and tenderness from her parents. More than her sister. She was very attached to her mother, and when her mom was away for only a few hours, she would wait for her in front of the house with tears running down her face. She was at peace only when her mom was finally home. Her calmness never lasted long, as she would always end up doing something to upset her parents. This caused her being grounded often and sometimes even physically scolded.

"This is why you are slim but with a nicely-shaped behind," I teased her, and she immediately showed disapproval. She did laugh, though.

At school and on the playground, she was tougher than the other kids, including boys who were older than her. She was in a good physical condition, always running, climbing, or hiking. Her slim body and gentle look surprised anyone that didn't know her yet. Eliza became soon the hero among the children in the vicinity by being the one that stopped a fire in some nearby bushes. She never told anyone that she was the one that accidentally started it. Even the most innocent children lie, don't they? She wasn't technically lying. She was just feeling ashamed and afraid to reveal many things about her, including starting the fire.

She had already kept many secrets from a young age. Secrets that I was yet to find out. *Drip, drip, drip.*

Eliza didn't like school during the first years. That is quite normal for a child. She found her classes boring, and she rather enjoyed running around the school yard during breaks. Her parents weren't too demanding regarding her education, so she lingered around average grades until the end of the 6$^{th}$ grade. You can say that the majority of kids don't like going to school.

Another thing that was different with me was that my parents were constantly checking on me and my siblings, making sure we studied, did our homework, and got good grades. I remember one day when I came home, happily telling my mom "I got the maximum grade on my test; will I get any money?" I only asked her for money because I had heard that many kids in my class were getting paid for their occasionally good grades. I constantly had good grades, and I thought I deserved the financial compensation.

"Are you learning for me or for yourself?" was my mom's reaction.

Was I learning for her? Of course not. So she made sure it was clear that we should learn for ourselves, for our own futures. I never asked for money again, but I didn't stop doing my best in school.

Eliza didn't have that kind of input from her parents. "Maybe I did, but I fully ignored them, so they gave up," she said. "I'm a really stubborn person," she added, with the normal smile that I became so used to.

In time, I would often notice that she is one of the most unyielding people I knew. At the beginning of the 7$^{th}$ grade, it was her determination and a new teacher that made her decide that she wanted to have good grades. "I like you. You are a smart one," said the teacher, and these short statements made Eliza finally believe in herself.

Her perseverance made her not only go from minimum grades to the maximum, but she was also participating and winning first prizes at county and national competitions for more than one subject. She surprised everyone, even herself. "I wanted to prove myself I was not stupid. Too many thought I was dumb, but luckily, not the new teacher," she added.

I hope that, by now, she knows that she is far from being stupid. She is one of the most intelligent people I know.

Some years later, still taking her studying seriously, she graduated and finished among the top GPAs in her year. Soon, she took on her first job as a social worker. Eliza's wish to help people, despite her social phobias, was huge. And I bet she is as good as a worker as she is as a friend and mother. The very best.

Eliza had friends. They were actually children from the neighborhood, and it was normal for them to play together. As she grew up during the time when the Internet was at its beginnings, playing outside was the main attraction for kids. Looking back, she feels that none of those old friends really knew her. Not even her older sister. An introvert. She was lazy regarding doing the household chores her mother assigned and learning during her first few years of school, but she was an ambitious person. She still is.

Keeping many things to herself was making her unapproachable. Sure, she could play games or go for a run, go swimming, or do some crazy stuff with other teens, but she hardly let anyone get close to her. Hence, she didn't get her first boyfriend until the age of eighteen. She met him during a period of time that she felt sad and lonely, and somehow, he had managed to make her open up a bit. She knew nothing about love and relationships. She simply went with the flow.

One year later, she became pregnant. It wasn't planned, and she wasn't even aware of it right away. It had been more than two months by the time she found out. At the beginning of the pregnancy, she won the local medal for the most talented woman football player. Yes, my friend was playing football[1] and "was the most promising young woman football player in the county," according to the newspapers.

I found this information out on the Internet later on. I was impressed and surprised she hadn't told me this herself. But Eliza is not the type of person to brag. She is actually too humble. A great quality rarely met but also another sign of lacking self-confidence.

At the age of eighteen, she was still practically a child, yet one to become a mother. Her boyfriend was shocked too by the news, and together, they decided what would be the next step. Luckily, Eliza's slim body and barely-noticed pregnancy helped them gain time until she was six months' pregnant.

She stopped playing football, but she never regretted doing so. The son she was about to give birth to was going to be her world, her love, her everything. And when that newborn baby smiled at her, she knew her life had a new meaning. Or better said, she finally discovered its meaning.

She knew very little about relationships and pregnancies. She decided not to go further with her studies, as she felt she wouldn't be able to manage raising a child, working a job, and studying for school all at once. She was still too young to cope with everything. Going to the university was initially the next step she had planned for herself. Everything was changing now. She wanted to prove that she was more capable

---

[1] American soccer.

## ADHD: LIFE IS BEAUTIFUL

than those that mocked her. The pregnancy wasn't helping, though. "One day, I will," she said.

While growing up, her good heart was often taken advantage of. It made a mark on her, and she didn't have the means or the strength to show everyone how wrong they were. Living in a small town and being young with a child were not easy to handle. People started to gossip, and Eliza was really affected by all of it. She hoped, though, that one day, she'd have the chance to shut their mouths. She was indeed sensitive. But the life inside her was giving her new strength. When she told me about this part of her life, I felt a deep feeling of admiration growing.

I know that many young girls in her situation would think about or be advised to give up on their pregnancy. She didn't. And she never regretted it. Not even for a second. Not even when her parents refused to help her when they found out. Not even when she was fighting with depression after many sleepless nights of taking care of her newborn baby and worrying about the future. Despite her gentle heart, unreasonable low self-esteem, and shyness, Eliza is a strong person.

# 4
## My Sweet, Angry Friend

*Drip, drip, drip,* and then there was silence.

I didn't find out what happened with the boyfriend, if they got married, or where he was. I only got the idea that he wasn't present in their life anymore, or at least not every day. I didn't get a verbal answer when I asked. I was getting used to that. It was the expression on her face, a mix of sadness and determination, followed by a sheepish smile that gave me a hint. And this is exactly the most common expression Eliza has on her face — that is, when she is not laughing.

I was becoming more aware how lucky I was to have tremendously supportive parents and to not have to face the tough situations Eliza had to put up with. How could her parents be so mean? Too many sad things are happening in the world. Family should be that one thing that you can count on. Why did they refuse to offer her that? My head was full of unanswered questions. In time, all of them would be clarified. I eventually also realized that, good or bad, everything was meant to happen. Everything played its role.

"Where were you when your parents refused to help you?" I asked, wondering at the same time who was babysitting while she was with me. We were having coffee on a terrace with a sea view. Hearing her life story made me forget where I was. The sound of the people enjoying the beach was muted by everything I was hearing. Only when I saw her moving her gaze towards the sea, not facing me, did I become aware again of reality. I thought I had a stressful life, but boy, listening to her story made me think all my problems were nothing.

"I was staying at my sister's place for a while."

"And how are things with your parents now?"

"My mom is living at my place." Her answer surprised me, and I'm sure I couldn't hide it.

"I thought you weren't in contact anymore."

"We are not on the best terms, but she is not a bad person. I tried to understand her. I will never forget what she did, but I managed, over time, to forgive her. I wasn't a perfect kid either."

I was not surprised at all. I knew already that Eliza had a big heart and that family connections are supposed to be strong enough to go over bigger things. Still, I wish her mother would have reacted differently back then.

"Looking back, I think it helped me. You know… what she did. I had to hit the real bottom in order to rise."

"Like a Phoenix," I said, and she laughed. I loved her laugh even more than her sweet, sheepish smile.

"Why is she living at your place? Where is your dad? I'm sorry if I'm being too nosy."

"It's a long story," she said, and she stopped.

I knew that could mean that it will take maybe a few more hangouts before I'd get to learn more. She surprised me, though, when she actually continued.

"Due to their health issues, my sister and I decided to take care of them. Our mother lives at my place, and our father, at hers. They are divorced and don't work anymore, so they can't afford a place on their own."

"Isn't it ironic that they need you now?"

"Yeah, you could look at it like that. It is still good for me. She loves Peter, and I do often need a babysitter. Peter is very particular, and he wouldn't be easy to handle. And he's very picky regarding food. He eats only what my mother cooks."

"What do you mean by 'particular'? I found him to be really sweet and easygoing."

"Yes, he is sweet. You have seen him only few times, though, so you don't know how he can be. I love him, but at times, he drives me crazy."

"I still believe he is sweet. A bit hyperactive, but fun to be with. What child isn't hyperactive, after all?"

"Hahaha. Yes, he is excessively active."

I smiled not because I thought she said something funny but because her laughing felt contagious.

Eliza suddenly answered her phone. "Hello? Yes, I'm coming. Bye."

"We have to go," she said in a hurry, already looking for the waiter so she could pay the bill.

"Already? I thought we were going to go swimming now," I said, a bit disappointed.

"We will, but I need to go pick up Peter first. I promised him that we would go to the beach after lunch."

"Oh, cool. I'm looking forward to spend a day on the beach with him."

"We shall see," she said, winking while unlocking the car. Her tanned body was already inside, music playing loudly while I barely managed to open my door. The next moment, the wheels squealed, and I looked back and convinced myself they left a mark on the asphalt. The sound caught everyone's attention. Looking at her, I saw she was smiling. It was the other side of her now. She changed from the calm, sensible, and fragile woman into an adrenaline-junkie, everything-to-the extreme one.

"I can't wait to see him. To kiss his sweet little hands. Oh, how much I miss him."

Not having children of my own, I couldn't understand how you could miss them so much after only one hour. I know now that this is true for her. The older Peter got, the more she missed him, which made it harder to stay apart from him. At times, I thought it was an addiction. Later, I would discover the real reason.

The day was about to continue differently. Peter joined us. He was now six-and-a-half.

He occupied his car-seat in the back of the car. He barely waved or showed any sign that he acknowledged that I was there. I tried to have a conversation with him, but he was too occupied with a game on Eliza's phone. Even after Eliza tried to force him to talk to me, he didn't behave much differently. He continued playing. I glanced over my shoulder every so often, and I saw him fully concentrated on an *Angry Birds* game. And he did look like an angry bird each time something got on his nerves. *'He is still sweet, a sweet angry bird,'* I told myself.

It was a Saturday, the weather was perfect for swimming, and the beach was pretty crowded with tourists and locals. We managed to find a place in the shade and put down our stuff. I was thrilled to be with them on the beach. I knew it was going to be different from our previous hangouts, but I had no idea to what extent.

At the speed of light and an unimaginable eagerness, Peter was already in the water. He was swimming, splashing everyone around him, going in and out of the water every two minutes, jumping, and making lots of happy sounds. I had a fun time even when I was just observing him. I changed into my bathing suit and entered the clear blue sea closer to Peter.

"Will you keep an eye on him?" Eliza asked me, because she was planning to go for a long swim. I nodded, and she took off. I only looked at her shortly and noticed her in the distance, moving like a professional swimmer. I wished I could swim like that. I was an amateur swimmer, always keeping close to the shore. I felt safer that way.

For a few minutes, I could keep Peter's interest and could play with him in the water, but it was obvious that I wasn't entertaining enough. He got bored and swam away. Close by, there was a group of people playing water polo. Committed to my assignment, I watched him. I saw him swimming distinctly in their direction. He went directly between them. His little head could be seen close to the goalkeeper or among the rest of the players. Where there were more of them, he was there, too. He was smiling, laughing, and full of excitement. A really cheeky kid.

The players were adults and didn't say anything to him. At one point, the ball reached him, and he started swimming away, pushing the ball in the direction outside of their imaginary game field.

"Peter, give back the ball," I yelled. I don't know if he heard me or not, but he was laughing and swimming even faster now in his chosen direction. The guys watching Peter stopped laughing, but none of them swam towards him or said anything.

"Go return the ball," I told him the moment I was close enough to him.

"Look what I have." He proudly showed the ball to me.

"It is not yours, Peter, so why did you take it?" I said, feeling a bit upset.

"They were all throwing it around, so I thought 'finders-keepers,'" he answered joyfully.

"It is their ball. Return it now!" I said authoritatively, but it seemed that he didn't understand me. In time, I would better speak his language, but I was still having issues, so I thought he couldn't understand me properly.

"Did you understand what I said?" I asked him, lowering my voice.

"Yes," he answered, his eyes pointed down.

I tried to explain to him what it was they were playing. He seemed to understand that it wasn't right to do what he did, so he handed me the ball, and I threw back to the guys. They continued playing. Peter continued his fun in the water, and I was again swimming sort of peacefully, always with my face towards him. From a distance, I could see Eliza's hands moving like a pro. She was still far away from us.

The next moment, I noticed Peter wasn't in my view anymore. Agitated, I started looking around, trying to distinguish his little, wet, blond-curled head, but he was nowhere to be seen. There were too many children around, and the strong sun reflecting on the water and blurring my vision was not helping. I started panicking.

"Peter! Peter!" I yelled. I wasn't loud enough to be heard over the sound of all the kids playing and swimming in the area. I went deeper into the water, constantly looking. I tried to calm myself: *'He is fine. Don't panic. He is a good swimmer and couldn't have gone too far. I lost sight of him for only a second.'*

Words didn't help. The relief came only when I finally spotted him. He was again between the water polo players, making turns and splashing everyone that came close to him. It made me smile to see how he didn't think he would be a bother to them and that he wasn't afraid that they may say something to him. He was a little boy; they were big men with strong muscles. He was having fun. I managed, though, to get his attention and called him to come over to me. I felt relieved, but I was angry at him.

"Why did you go over there again? Can you please try swimming closer to me so I can see you?" I asked in a serious tone.

"'K," was his answer, which I supposed meant he understood what I'd asked of him. The following five minutes were eventless. He was swimming around me, going under the water on one side, coming out on the other. Each time he came out of the water, he yelled, "Nickelodeon." I was calm again, so I found it amusing. I knew already from Eliza that he was a huge fan. I noticed some looks from the adults and children around that showed that they didn't seem to think it was so sweet, but I didn't bother.

"What do we have to eat?" he asked.

"I have some peaches in my bag. Do you want one?"

"Uh, yuck!" was his answer, which I didn't expect.

"Don't you like peaches?"

"No."

"Which fruits do you like?"

"I like potatoes."

"Potatoes aren't fruits."

"Potatoes are the best, especially fries from McDonald's."

I decided not to comment. What did I know about children anyway?

"Do we have potato chips?"

"I don't know. Let's wait for your mom."

"'K," he answered. He was clearly unhappy. A second later, he said, "I am thirsty."

"Is water good?" I decided to check, rather than dig something out for him that he wouldn't drink.

"I want Coca-Cola."

"Coca-Cola isn't healthy, Peter."

"Yes it is. I want Coca-Cola and potato chips." He seemed to have a bit of fun with me, as I was losing patience. More proof that I didn't have much experience with kids.

"I only have water," I answered, still a bit on edge.

"'K." I guess he was really thirsty for even water to be fine.

"Can you go look in my bag and get the bottle of water out?" I felt a bit lazy for not getting up and fetching it myself. And I had no idea that it would have been smarter if I would have gone with him. As I was carrying minimal luggage during my weekends to the seaside, I was using my rucksack instead of a handbag and had everything in there: documents, money, and lots of other stuff.

I watched him getting out of the water and his slim body making small and fast steps towards our parasols. Well, at first, he was heading towards the wrong one, but I pointed him in the right direction. He picked up the rucksack, asking me from a distance if that was the right one. I confirmed, and then he placed it down, turned his back to me, and a couple of minutes later, I saw him drinking. Problem solved.

He came back and continued doing his now-familiar exhibitions. He did have lots of energy, and doing the same movement for more than thirty seconds seemed to bore him. I looked at the other children, and they all seemed to move, play, and talk in slow motion, compared to Peter. After some time, Eliza finished her long swim and came closer to us. She got out of the sea and lay down on the beach close to us. I decided to join her. Eliza's eyes were constantly on Peter. Babysitting time was over for me. I could relax now.

# 5
## Nickelodeon Rules

I looked around, lost in my thoughts. I decided to lie down on the small stones. I didn't even need to go and pick up my book. I was admiring the blue sky instead. There wasn't even one cloud in it. Many seagulls were flying around. I watched them with a grin on my face. I was flying with them. I was landing on the water and taking off again towards the sky. I was getting lost in time. I wasn't paying attention to the passing minutes. I wasn't thinking of the things that usually occupied my thoughts. I didn't need a book that would draw me into its pages. I was just simply enjoying the moment. A moment of nothingness. Yet, a moment of fullness.

The loud, shrill, droning noise of the cicadas from the nearby pine trees was soothing. Normally, similar sounds would drive me nuts. But not today. A gentle breeze was caressing my body. Everything was so relaxing. Why don't I do this at home? Why don't I take few minutes for myself? It doesn't have to be close to the sea; my city was far from it anyway. It could be enough just to be somewhere in the fresh air, to lie on the grass or on a bench and look at the sky. The sky is beautiful everywhere.

It wasn't only the sky, though. To me, that day, it meant much more. It felt as if this moment here was made for me. I knew now why Eliza enjoyed doing this so much. Being quiet. Shutting out the rest of the world. Living in the moment. I couldn't manage to do this in the past. If not my body, my mind was constantly working on something. Present, future, past. Nothing was important now. It was just this moment, lost in time.

I was starting to understand what she had already been trying to tell me on several occasions. I told her stories about my life at the beginning, so she knew a lot about me. In time, she started to believe too that the real "me" was here in this place. One needle-like leaf fell on my belly. I became aware again of what was happening around me. But still happy, content, relaxed.

Peter was closer. He was standing, the water level a bit above his waist and he was splashing around, moving his hands back and forth, and then making pirouettes, and jumping. At one moment, it seemed he was fighting with an invisible something, hitting the water with his fists and making sounds of victory. The other children were keeping a distance from him. It was his show.

"He is in his movie now," Eliza explained laughing.

"What kind of movie? Like a cartoon that he enjoys?" I asked.

"I don't know. Look at him. He acts as if he's fighting some enemies."

We both continued watching him.

"Nickelodeon" came out of his mouth a few moments later.

"Nickelodeon sucks," said a boy with a stronger body that seemed to be older than him.

"What?" said a now-angry Peter. "Nickelodeon rules!" he yelled.

He approached the guy and started splashing him. He was so determined in his action and so affected by the other child's statement that he didn't care that he was overpowered. He also seemed not to acknowledge right away that Eliza was telling him to stop. He did stop, though. It was when the other child decided to go away. A big grin showed on Peter's face. He won. Yes, he was a true Nickelodeon fan.

"Mama, do we have chips?" he asked from a distance.

"Yes, we do."

"Yay!"

He came out running, and the three of us headed towards our parasols.

"What happened here?" Eliza asked. I was behind her, so it took me a second to see for myself. The whole content of my rucksack was spread around. It was everything: money, documents, cell phone, lipstick, and, among other things, tampons spread everywhere. I was sure I had packed them in a small, zipped toiletries bag.

"Peter!" I yelled, this time not because I panicked, but because I was furious. "Why did you do this?" I asked crossly while placing all my stuff back where it belonged.

"I was searching for water."

"In this little bag?" I yelled, shoving all the tampons inside.

"I don't know," he said, looking at the pebbles instead of me.

"Why did you have to go through everything?" I just couldn't calm myself. The moment of serenity from before was gone. Past. Forgotten. I was in the present and allowed myself to get annoyed over a childish thing.

"Tell Nico that you are sorry," Eliza told him in a blank voice. She didn't sound fully on my side. I get it, it was her son, and I shouldn't allow myself to get so nerve-wracked.

I looked at Peter, and it was clear he was affected, but he said nothing. It wasn't such a bad thing after all. I felt awful for raising my voice at him, and I also didn't know how Eliza was taking this.

I decided I should apologize for my exaggerated reaction and tone of voice. She started laughing while wiping his body with a towel.

"Do you still think he is sweet?"

I took a moment and looked at Peter, at his wet, blond curls and his long eye-lashes that covered his big, beautiful blue eyes. His gaze was still facing the ground, and it seemed that he was crying.

"I'm sorry, Peter. I didn't mean to be so harsh on you," I said apologetically.

Yep, he was crying, and went in Eliza's arms to hide from me.

"I was only searching for the bottle of water," he whispered.

"Shh, it's okay, baby, don't cry."

I honestly regretted my reaction. I had no idea that it would affect him so much. On the other hand, I don't think I could have reacted differently, but I would know better in the future.

"Will you forgive me?" I asked while trying to hold his hand.

He pulled it away immediately and sunk even deeper into Eliza's hug.

I heard him whispering something but couldn't understand what he was saying.

"You need to say out loud 'Nickelodeon rules' if you want him to forgive you," Eliza transmitted to me. She was smiling.

"What? This is silly." It wasn't going to happen.

Nope. It wasn't silly for Peter. He really meant it. He didn't speak with me directly until much later. Not even when he was eating his favorite fries during our stop at McDonald's. But he did help by carrying not only my heavy rucksack but also part of the stuff we had at the beach. It was funny to see his determination in carrying everything. His slim, tiny body was stronger than it looked. Was he sending me some message with his gesture? I found this to be really sweet, and I didn't mind when few things fell out or when the towel was collecting dirt on the way. In his awkward way, he was probably showing that he was sorry for the trouble he had caused.

"He really doesn't want to talk to me," I told Eliza in awe when we were in the car again.

"Peter, that's enough. Be polite and talk to her. She is our friend, and we should treat our friends nicely."

"No, she was mean before. I was only looking for the water," he said, still kind of furious.

And I decided to do something that I never thought I would. "Nickelodeon rules!" I yelled with a smile, and Peter started laughing.

"Yay!"

I felt at ease again, and I smiled upon seeing the sparkles in his eyes.

A bit later, we have left Peter at home and Eliza drove me to my accommodations. On the way, I managed to tell her everything that happened during the only thirty minutes she was away swimming. She was laughing -- like a really good laugh.

"I know that Peter can be a bit boring with his Nickelodeon thing. But there are few things that he loves, and Nickelodeon is one of them. It requires a lot of energy to be a parent, especially if you are a single mom. I felt him very alive and kicking already before I gave birth. I couldn't sleep for months when he was born. I had to feed him constantly, and I really couldn't imagine that my little baby could really eat that much. Always active, always hungry, and, if not one of those, always crying. Still, he is my happiness. My sweet angry boy." She smiled and got lost into a pensive state during the next few minutes of driving.

"Thank you for a wonderful day and sorry once again for my reaction," I told her through the opened car window after I got out.

"Thank you, Nico, for spending time with us and... for not being judgmental." She left before I managed to ask or say anything in response.

Was she sending me a message in a subtle or passive-aggressive way, or did she really believe I wasn't judging them?

The night fell, and everything was again hushed and motionless. Before falling asleep in my bed, going over all the events of the day as I usually do, I realized that this day only had one bad thing. And that was my harsh reaction.

***

I managed to visit my friends a few more times that summer. The purpose of my visit wasn't to get away from my daily stressful life anymore. I was simply enjoying the time spent with them. We went to the beach on a few occasions, we went hiking, and we played football in a valley with a beautiful view across the sea and the hills, away from the city. Peter was getting used to me and felt comfortable in my presence, and I thought I was comfortable in his.

"Do you like Nickelodeon?" Peter asked each kid we were met on our long walk in a national park. Many people were walking in both directions. Peter was having his typical walk, never straight, always climbing on anything possible, and always yelling about or asking about Nickelodeon. I admit, because of him, I watched a bit of this TV station to have an idea what kind of shows they played. I was sure the majority of the parents would know it pretty well. So the parents we met on our walk were smiling at his questions, while the kids' reactions were different. Some of them were confirming, and Peter tried to talk more with them, but others were just saying an embarrassed "yes" and moving on. There were some that laughed at him. This made Peter momentarily sad, and he walked a bit further in silence.

"Hello."

"Hi."

"Good day."

These were the words adults were exchanging among each other.

"Do you know these people?" Peter asked me.

"No, but this is what people do. People greet each other when they pass by when in nature, hiking, or just walking like we are now," I explained.

"Hello," came shyly out of his mouth when we met the next people on our way. He continued doing so the whole way, giving the Nickelodeon thing a break.

He took my hand for the first time, and we walked together. I was telling him funny little stories or answering a million questions about everything that crossed his mind. I was surprised how many things he could actually understand. Eliza was more or less listening to and smiling at our conversations.

"I admire your patience," she told me at one point.

While I enjoyed talking to Peter, I did find it a bit exhausting, but nothing extreme. For me, it was a day or two spent together, while Eliza had to put up with his energy every day. She had lots of energy herself, so it probably was not so tiring for her.

We stopped at one area that had an amazing view over a beautiful lake surrounded by green small trees. We had our drinks. Peter's was of course Coca-Cola, which was something that his mom did allow from time to time. If you had asked him, he would have drunk only that. Water? Yuck. Coca-Cola? Yay!

We clinked our drinks, and what do you think we cheered for? Nickelodeon!

I laughed at Peter telling me that he was going to work for Nickelodeon when he turned 11. I didn't want to spoil his dreams, so I went along with the conversation, trying to understand how his mind functioned. I got his full attention when I told him I was going to write an email to the TV station.

And I did do that a few days later. I mentioned them that they have a big fan in Peter and that his birthday is coming up, and I asked them nicely if they could take their time and wish him happy birthday. Unfortunately, they never answered. But over time, Peter passed through this phase. He still watches his favorite TV station, but he has other things to talk about now.

Despite the fact that he was surprising me with intelligent comments and questions, he was still much more of a baby than other kids his age. But he had such a good, not corrupted heart. Maybe I was subjective. Maybe I had no knowledge of children. But I thought, and I still think, that Peter is a smart young boy. Eliza is the same, and both of them can be clumsy, moody, energetic, and fun.

"Do you like Nico?" Eliza asked her son that evening when we were returning from a splendid day spent among nature.

"Yes," said Peter while enjoying his ice cream cone. I saw the ice cream dripping all over his hands. I took out some napkins and wiped his hands with them. As he was a bit difficult to reach from the front seat, I handed him a napkin to wipe his face. He did, in his funny, clumsy way.

"Is Nico your friend?"

"Yes. Nico and Lara are my BFFs."

Wow. His words touched my heart. I had some competition, though.

"Who is Lara?"

"My cousin," he explained.

Well, I could live with that. These were, of course, funny, silly thoughts. It is, however, a pleasant feeling to hear that you are the best friend of someone, especially of a naughty but sweet little boy.

"Lara is great. You will meet her tomorrow," Eliza added.

And I did. Lara was the opposite of Peter. They were the same age, but she was silent while he talked loudly, a lot, and quite often. He was running fast while she wanted to take it slow. He was making fun of her while she simply just smiled at him, not at all bothered. She seemed to have lots of patience for all his moods, words, and actions. And it was obvious that Peter did care a lot for her. I could see some similarities between Lara and myself and thought that we may be the type of people that suited Peter. Eliza too. Still, I continued to be baffled that Peter didn't have too many friends. He seemed so enjoyable, playful, and fun to be with. I would find out the reasons for that later on.

The moments when Peter was part of our get-together, peacefulness was more of a rarity.

Lovely. Lively. Worrying. Energetic. Dynamic. Frustrating. Compelling. Amusing. Sadness. Laughter. Joy. Fun. Love. True friendship. These words would describe our time better. Even if some of them weren't on the positive side, the overall impression was a great one, with lots of patience and understanding on my part. Patience, I had. Acceptance and tolerance, I was yet to find some more with time.

# 6
## Are There Any Pigs in Italy?

Summer was slowly ending. On the beach, our escapades became less frequent, but the temperatures during early autumn by the seaside were perfect for long walks. They were a great way to enjoy nature. Occasionally, I did this alone, but mostly with my friends. I realized I was totally ignoring some other friends I'd also made there. This wasn't because they weren't nice people. Some of them were too preoccupied with money, jobs, and other day-to-day matters. I was also like this not so long ago, and I knew many similar people in my hometown.

I was simply enjoying my new companions more. They brought out a different side of my personality. This other me was more in touch with nature. I was learning, although a little late, that the real pleasures in life are not material possessions and hitting goals at work. This new part of me enjoyed the smell of a lavender field rather than the scent of the most expensive perfume.

I was now living for the moment, and one benefit of this was it helped me get through the other less pleasant times. I realized that real friends don't need to have everything in common. I believe that true friendship should be based on genuine feelings of understanding, acceptance, and bits and pieces of sharing thoughts and time with each other. The new me was learning to be more tolerant and accepting. I have failed at doing so in the past, but here, I was always learning from my mistakes.

Speaking of mistakes, I was about to make a big one.

"Do you like to travel?" I asked Eliza one day while driving to pick up Peter from home. It was a peaceful Sunday morning, and I still had a few more hours there. The three of us were planning to see one of the ancient fortresses overlooking the sea and the city.

"Yes, I do, but I've never traveled outside of the country."

"Oh, really?" That actually surprised me.

"It is not easy, taking care of Peter and working to support us. I'm trying to provide for him as best I can. I want him to have everything, but I have never had the time or spare money for foreign travel, but who knows? Maybe one day the chance will come." Despite her hope and optimism, there was a tone of sadness in her words.

As time passed, Eliza opened up more and more, and I saw less of the sheepish smile that had thus far been a constant during our conversations. She still brought it out each time we met almost anyone else. I was entering deeper in their circle of trust. I promised myself that I would never break it.

"If you could go anywhere in the world, where would it be?" I asked, already dreaming about the many destinations on my own bucket list.

"Amsterdam, the Netherlands," she replied instantly, with a sparkle in her eyes.

"Let's go there then."

"When?" she asked, clearly surprised, but I could see excitement in her eyes.

"I don't know. As soon as we both have a gap at the same time in our schedules."

She considered the proposal for a while. "It will have to wait," she said. Her eyes had lost their excitement.

"Why? If it's due to money, I can help," I offered, already thrilled at the thought of the two of us going on a trip someplace other than her home city and its surroundings.

"I can't be away from Peter for more than a day." She was sincere, and I tried to understand.

"Let's take him too."

"As much as I would love for him to see the world, I don't think he'd enjoy it too much, and I'm sure you wouldn't enjoy it at all."

"I'm sure we can find things to entertain him as well," I said, convinced that I was right, although I had no concrete ideas.

"You still don't know him," she smiled, amused.

"I think I do."

"You don't know him enough. It's okay. I don't blame you." Her mood was changing by the second. It felt like a constant conflict of emotions and thoughts inside her head battling each other. Sometimes, she was full of desire and excitement over the possibility of something new, but then, reality would return and spoil it, bringing her down. Maybe she was hiding behind mental barriers. Maybe something could be done.

My mind was working fast, and I came up with another proposal. I was sure that an amusement park could be the perfect destination for the three of us.

"What about a trip to Gardaland, Italy?"

"It sounds like fun, but I'm still not sure."

"What kid wouldn't like that?" I was persistent.

"I don't think you understand that taking a trip can get unpleasant at times, no matter how exciting you think it might be."

"How about you check with Peter? Show him the park's website and let him decide," I offered.

"Yes. That's a deal," she said, looking a little happier this time.

"This will be perfect. I see no reason why a child wouldn't enjoy spending a day in an amusement park. I'm sure he'll love it." How little I knew.

Soon after, we picked up Peter.

"Hello, Peter," I said cheerfully.

"Hey," he greeted me back without reciprocating my excitement. Then he was quiet. During the rest of the journey, he was totally immersed in his game, although he also appeared to be gradually getting a little more nervous. The repetitive noises of his game were annoying, but I knew better than to mention this.

"Turn the volume down, Peter." Eliza yelled at him.

Even though it seemed too loud, he didn't react.

"Stop that game now, or I will take the phone." After few more shouts from Eliza, Peter finally listened and stopped playing. He stared through the car window. I wondered what thoughts were passing through that little curly-haired head of his.

"Where are we going?" he asked after quickly becoming bored.

"Up on the hill to the fortress."

"Oh, no! That is so dull. Why can't I just stay at home and play my game? I was just about to reach the next level when you stopped me. Who knows when I am going to reach it now?"

I smiled at his passionate interest in *Angry Birds*, but it was clear that to him, this was not at all funny. We stuck to our plan, though.

During the climb, he was constantly zigzagging along the path, and he didn't seem to want to talk. He held in his hand a plush toy red bird. He had told me previously the names of all the birds from both his game and cartoon, but I couldn't remember any of it.

I found out, though, that due to the game, he had now started to love pigs. Funny, considering that the pigs in the game seem to have a negative role. The little pinkish-white piggy was his favorite animal. He was the first child I'd ever known to want a pig as a pet. Talking with him about an imaginary piggy cheered him up. He'd sometimes make funny pig sounds, and he'd be hilarious then, but today, he wasn't in that kind of mood.

We managed to reach the top, and we stopped for a while to enjoy the view. I think I was the only one that enjoyed it, as Eliza was always watching Peter, as he was constantly moving close to the edge of the field, and it would have been dangerous if he had slipped. The more she asked him to move away from the edge, the closer he got. I started to worry too. He seemed to not understand our concern and continued walking almost like a gymnast on a narrow bar in an awkward way.

Eliza stopped yelling at him but stayed close, with one hand on his, ensuring she could react in time if necessary.

"Come here, Peter. I want to tell you something important." Luckily, this was the thing that finally made him give up on the hazardous balancing act. Or maybe he just got bored of what he was doing, typical for Peter.

"What?" he said, not quite convinced that he would be too interested in what I was about to say.

"What would you say if, one day, we were to visit an amusement park?"

"What is that?" he asked.

"Something similar to the Luna Park that comes to your city with the water toboggans you enjoy during the summer, but much bigger and with lots of other fun entertainment for kids."

"Where is that?" He sounded enthusiastic.

"It is in another country."

"What country?"

"Italy."

"Where is that?"

"You will learn in school soon."

"I don't want to go to school." His mood changed again.

"You'll have lots of fun there, Peter. You'll see."

"I don't think so." He was so sure, yet he didn't have a clue what school was like.

"School may be cool too; believe me."

He didn't look convinced.

"Forget about the school now. Let me tell you more about this country and its amusement park."

I tried to tell him that there were many countries in the world, and one of them was his. I added that each country has lots of interesting places and lots of cool stuff for kids. He listened carefully and seemed to be absorbing the information. At times, he seemed a bit confused, as if he weren't expecting that there were cities with higher populations than his, but slowly, he was processing everything. He became calm.

"How many hours will we be there?" he asked.

"We will need at least two or three days altogether."

He looked sad. "That's too long. I will miss Grandma. I don't want to go."

It was sweet. I did my best and tried to convince him that Grandma will miss him too, but she would also be happy for him. She would want her favorite grandson to have a good time and see new things.

"'Kay" was his delayed response. "Do they have pigs in Italy?" he asked with slightly more enthusiasm.

"Yes, they do, but I don't know if we will meet any." I couldn't hide my smile. I looked at Eliza, who was carefully listening to our conversation.

"I'm sure we will. Let's go then." He turned to Eliza. "Mom, when can we go?"

If I could have, I would have taken him then and there. He was adorable in all his enthusiasm, probably not because of Gardaland but because of the pigs.

During the hours that followed, Gardaland was our only topic of conversation. They eventually took me to the bus station. It was, sadly, time for me to leave. Peter was watching the buses that were waiting for their passengers to embark.

"Goodbye, Peter," I said, when I managed to grab his attention. He turned to me, and for the first time, he hugged me goodbye and kissed my cheek. He did this in his awkward, childish manner, but it was the sweetest goodbye I'd ever received. I turned to Eliza, and her eyes looked moist with tears. It was only at this moment that I realized my eyes were welling up with tears too as I boarded the bus. These were tears of joy and a feeling of love growing for this sweet, innocent boy.

"We must plan this Gardaland trip as soon as possible," said a text from Eliza one hour later. "I showed Peter the pictures and videos on the Internet, and he was so excited." Another message followed half an hour later: "Nico, you have to make the time to go to Gardaland. He can't stop talking about it. I'll have no peace until I take him there."

I smiled, and I answered back that I will do my best to plan the trip and find time as soon as possible.

Five days later, I did exactly that. Before he started school, we would take Peter to Gardaland. My first trip ever with a child. Their first trip out of the country. I was in charge of organizing and arranging everything not only because I had experience traveling but also because Eliza didn't have the patience to deal with the details. She had no problem driving, and I enjoyed being a passenger and planning trips, and navigation with a map was my specialty. *'Yin and yang,'* I thought again.

As per my plan, we set off early in the morning. Eliza told me that Peter didn't want to go to bed on time the previous night because he was too excited about the trip. His first long trip. We had almost eight hours of driving, and luckily, he slept for most of it. I thought, *'Traveling with a child is so easy.'*

However, problems soon started. During what was supposed to be a time of fun, excitement, and enjoyment, I had failed. As a friend and as a human. Looking back, I'm not proud of myself, but in mitigation, I have since changed my perspective and behavior, so I have forgiven myself a little.

## ADHD: LIFE IS BEAUTIFUL

We reached our accommodations in a small Italian city close to Gardaland. Our visit to the amusement park was to be on the following day. First, we wanted to see what this little city had to offer, have a proper meal and go to sleep early so we can be fully rested and energized for the next day.

Although walks among nature never seemed to be a problem for Peter, on this occasion, he whined and complained with every step. He took no interest in any of the buildings and places we passed. Eliza appeared to appreciate and admire everything. Luckily, we found a playground where we let Peter play for a few hours. His enthusiasm returned.

"I don't know where we are. I don't understand the language of these people here," I heard Peter telling his grandmother over the phone. She was missing him already, and that was understandable.

"I miss you too," he said. It was really touching to hear him say those words.

At one point, we told him about different countries and languages, but he didn't seem to care.

"You told me that pigs made the same sound everywhere. Why can't people speak the same?"

I was baffled, and all I could do was just laugh. He didn't think it was funny.

When we returned to our hotel, his disappointment continued. There was no cable TV, hence no Nickelodeon. I found another children's TV program, but it was in Italian. When we decided that it was time to turn off the lights and go to sleep, he wanted to play his game instead.

"I am not tired," he kept saying.

At first, Eliza had patience and let him stay up for several pleadings for "ten more minutes," but then, even she lost patience with him.

"I miss Grandma. I miss my room. I want to go home," Peter said when we finally called it a night.

"Aren't you happy that you will have a full day of fun tomorrow?" I asked.

"No," he snapped back.

"I would have been so happy if I'd had the chance to visit this park when I was your age," I added. I was surprised, as I didn't expect a child to be so underwhelmed about it. What had become of that enthusiasm flying out of him the other day?

"I don't care. I want to go home," he said blankly.

"You have no idea, Peter, how many kids would love to be in your place. We came here especially for you." Eliza was trying to help me.

"I don't care," he said repeatedly.

"That's enough, Peter." With this, Eliza managed to quiet him.

Later, she told me that it was very hard for him to be separated from his home environment. Every little change caused him stress. Still, she believed this would be fun for him, hoping he would adapt quickly.

# 7
## Gardaland

Nope, Gardaland wasn't for him. He didn't enjoy it — I have to give him that. But it wasn't for Eliza either.

"Why did you take us here?" both of them were saying after we finished our ride on the *Mammut* roller coaster. I had no idea they would get so scared. I only suggested it after Peter's million requests to go on Magic Mountain, and I thought that the *Montaigne-rouse* would have been too much for him.

"I didn't like it," they both said in unison.

It didn't bother me much with Eliza, since she was an adult. I managed to brighten Peter's mood a little after buying him some delicious gelato. We walked through the park, and he seemed to enjoy it and even wanted to try some other things. However, he had no patience for waiting in the long lines. He was constantly moaning, constantly complaining. His only non-complaining moments were during the 30 seconds or 1 minute we were on a ride and maybe for a minute after.

Then, he would say repeatedly:
"Why do we have to wait this long?"
"Why are so many people here?"
"Why won't they let us in?"
"Let's go in front."
"This is stupid."
"I want to go home."

At first, I had patience and tried to distract him or calm him down. We both did. We tried to entertain him with different games and funny stories while waiting in the queues. It didn't help.

Eliza lost her patience before I did. I resisted a bit longer but almost lost it when it was time for lunch. I could understand that children are picky regarding food. I was a picky person myself. Peter typically ate only potato chips and certain sweets. Yes, he could eat plenty of those. We didn't have any choice but buy him potato chips in the first restaurant that we'd managed to find with an empty table.

Close to us was a trampoline. Peter went to it immediately, with French fries in his hands. No matter how many times we told him that he should sit down quietly and eat, he wouldn't listen. Every now and then, he would come to pick up more fries, have a sip of Coke, and then go back. He seemed happier on the trampoline than on any of the other attractions.

Children were not allowed to have food on the trampoline, and the other parents were now giving us disapproving looks. Reacting quickly, Eliza managed to return Peter to our table.

She was angry. He was angry. I was disappointed.

I couldn't believe we had to leave the park prior to closing time. I was made to feel as if we were keeping him there by force. We headed back to our accommodations, and then, we took him once more to the small playground close by. He played alone, going on each item of equipment, one after another. None of them managed to hold his interest for more than a minute, but still, he did burn off some of his energy, moving from item to item, again and again.

We were sitting on the bench and watching him. Neither of us seemed very pleased about how the day had gone. We stopped talking. Eliza seemed lost in her thoughts too. It wasn't the same kind of pleasant silence that we had previously shared. It was a deliberate decision not to share our thoughts, as they could be hurtful, at least from my side.

I was expecting Peter to laugh and enjoy the whole day. It didn't happen. He, however, loved this simple playground, similar to the one he had at home, rather than all the amazing attractions in Gardaland. Here, he was alone. He didn't have to wait in queues. There was no annoying screaming. He seemed full of energy, yet content and peaceful.

We made a quick trip to get a pizza later on. This was just for Eliza and me. Peter would say, "That's yuck." Not only did his comments spoil our meal, but he also constantly moved his feet under the table, dropped stuff on the floor, spilled his juice, and played his game on the phone with the sound at full volume.

"Peter! Please stop fidgeting."

It felt as if everybody in the restaurant was looking at us. They were judging us. He looked at me with a shocked expression; Eliza looked away but said nothing. Had I been too sharp? Maybe. I'd lost it; that was for sure.

We ate as fast as we could and headed off to our hotel. I was frustrated but also felt bad for putting Peter in his place. He didn't enjoy being told off, and he was probably hungry. But he didn't want anything that was on the menu. Luckily, Eliza had some banana and yogurt with her, and she almost forced Peter to eat a little once were back in our room. I would often hear him say, "I'm never hungry," and I wondered why this kid wasn't just skin and bones, considering how little, and sometimes how poorly and infrequently, he ate.

Once bedtime arrived, the scenario as per the previous night was repeated. This time, I took the phone from Peter's hand and told him to go to sleep, turning off the lights without even asking Eliza. My nerves were seriously on edge. My head hurt despite the painkillers I'd taken earlier.

The next morning, we were due to travel back home. This meant another long day of driving. We needed sleep. I also needed a little peace of mind. This trip proved to be slightly too much for me. Eliza was right. Why hadn't I listened to her when she'd told me it wasn't going to be an easy trip with Peter? Why did he have no patience? He often ignored everything we said to him. Our words often just didn't seem to reach him. I loved Peter, but it was different to spend a few hours with him than it was to spend a few days. These two days seemed to have lasted forever. I thought about the next day and the likelihood that it would be similarly tiring. That wasn't helping.

The throbbing inside my head was now getting worse. I massaged my right temple, trying to relieve some of the inflammation. It felt a little better. The room was, thankfully, quiet. They both fell asleep quickly while I lay there, tossing and turning. I kept checking the time. I knew this silence would only last until the morning. Eventually, I managed to doze off and put to sleep my negative thoughts for a couple of hours.

The morning came. We barely had time for breakfast, and I couldn't afford to enjoy my drink from the café in peace within it. Instead, I had coffee to-go. The other guests in the café were giving us strange looks due to his peculiar mood. Peter was thrilled that we were returning home, and we had to pack the car quickly to stop him from becoming overexcited. It was clear that Gardaland and the whole trip so far had been more like torture, instead of fun, to Peter.

I was still a little angry but also trying to understand how it was for him. All we wanted was for him to have fun. That had been our only intention. All he wanted was Nickelodeon, his grandma, and the comfort of his room. He was probably too young to take pleasure in this kind of trip. He definitely didn't enjoy this. Eliza didn't enjoy it either. Me? I was already thinking, *'Why did I come up with the idea of taking this trip?'* But again, I kept those negative thoughts to myself.

Despite the fact that Peter was getting closer to home as each minute passed, he still continued to grumble and moan. This only stopped when he was permitted to play the game on his phone. Then we would be treated to a momentary pause in the screaming, complaining, and shifting about in the back seat. It was a great relief, but sadly, it didn't last long, as the battery soon died. Too soon. I had been enjoying the peace.

"When will we arrive home?"

"I didn't see any pigs. You said that there are pigs here too."

"How far must we drive now?"

"Mama, drive faster."

"Why are the cars in front of us driving so slowly?"

I stopped trying to answer him eventually. It felt as though whatever I said didn't make any difference. Peter was repeating all of the above, along with a few other comments not appropriate for a child. He did this almost every minute. I nearly managed to get his attention with some stories or bits of conversation, but all I was really doing was distracting him. I was becoming stressed out as well.

"I told you" seemed to be written on Eliza's expression when I managed to catch eye contact with her. Or maybe her silence meant something else. Peter was a really demanding child. I admired her for having the energy. I'd lost mine in less than two days with him. Although he was still cute in appearance, I started to like him less. I found him really annoying with his never-ending requests, constant interruptions, and lack of patience. This was happening almost every second.

"Peter, would you please shut up? I can't take it anymore," I yelled. Even louder than when I had to say "Nickelodeon rules." The little bit of patience that I had left lasted this long.

He did shut up. Probably because he was so surprised to hear me raising my voice. Eliza looked at me, and I couldn't understand what her expression meant.

"I'm sorry, Eliza. I know he is your child and that I don't have the right to yell at him, but he's driving me crazy."

She said nothing.

We drove in silence from that moment on. I was furious. I was like Peter now, anxious to arrive home. This wasn't my comfort zone either. Despite my high expectations, I didn't enjoy the trip. None of us did.

"I'm sorry you didn't have a nice time with us," the silence was interrupted by Eliza's words as I exited the car.

"Bye" was the only word I could say, barely able to look her in the eye.

I turned my back as fast as I could and left. I felt like crying out of disappointment, nerves, and frustration.

It could have been such a fun trip, but it wasn't. It wasn't fun for any of us, and worse still, this had maybe put an end to our friendship. I wasn't sure if I needed this kind of mental pressure in my life. I had enough stress already with my job and everything else.

My time here, changing the routine, was supposed to be the one in which to charge my batteries. I felt heartbroken, realizing that this will be the first time I had gone back with such negative feelings. I didn't like it. I didn't like anything. When I turned on the TV before sleeping, just to help me expel my negative thoughts, it was on Nickelodeon. I now hated Nickelodeon!

What was I turning into? Where was the new better me that I'd been discovering here? Why was Peter like that? Was it because he was too spoiled? I could imagine that being raised by a loving mom and grandmother, he would always get his way. Luckily, he shall be starting school soon. Maybe he will learn some discipline. Hopefully, he shall behave a little nicer. Maybe he will learn to be patient. Perhaps then, he will start living in reality and not in his baby-like fantasy like kids much younger than his age. Many "maybes," but one thing was for sure: I was not meant to have children. I don't have the required patience.

Sleep didn't come easy. I tossed and turned. I barely managed to close an eye for one hour during the whole night. I was exhausted mentally and physically.

The next day, I went home. I didn't call Eliza. She didn't call me either. Maybe this would be the end of our friendship.

\*\*\*

If I could turn back time, I would have done things differently. I would have tried to control my reactions. I would have tried to be more tolerant. I would have shown a better understanding of the situation. I wouldn't have had so many wrong moral judgments.

I know that Eliza thanked me once for not being judgmental, but that was then. What was she thinking now? Had I failed her? Had I failed our friendship?

# 8
# Who Invented School?

"I hate school" was the first thing Peter said one day in a phone conversation. It was our first communication over the phone since the trip. I knew he was supposed to start school that fall, but I didn't know how this had played out. Eliza and I had exchanged only a few texts since our trip, and these had not gone into great detail about our lives.

"Everything will be fine, Peter. Just give it some time," I said patiently, feeling sorry for him.

"I have to stay in my seat during class. Each time I stand, the teacher yells at me," he complained.

"I'm sure that can't be so bad. You will get used to it."

"It is bad. I don't want to go to school. I don't want to do any homework. I just want to play." He was sweet while saying that. I felt for him.

"Tell Nico what the teacher asked you today," Eliza said in the background, her tone amused.

"Oh, yes. The teacher asked all of us to name three friends, and when it was my turn, I said: Angry Birds, SpongeBob, and Oliver."

He was serious, but I couldn't help but laugh.

"Why are you laughing? I don't get it. Everyone in my class laughed too when I said that," he said unhappily.

"Well, because it's funny, Peter. You have named two cartoon friends. She meant real friends," I said calmly.

"But they are my real friends!" he shouted.

"I believe you, Peter. But they are only friends in virtual reality. Well, except for Oliver."

"Actually, Oliver is less of a friend, I realized today. He sits with me in the class, but he didn't mention me among his friends. I will forgive him."

The sincerity in his voice touched my heart. "I'm sure Oliver does think of you as a friend, but he has more than three, which is why he didn't mention you."

"Yes, I think so," he said, sounding happier.

We spoke a little longer, and then, he put Eliza on the phone.

"Hi, Nico. I'm sorry we haven't been in touch recently, but now with school starting, my day is packed. You can't believe how much homework they give in the first grade."

"I understand. Don't worry. In time, you will get into a routine."

"So, what do you think about Peter's friends? He still lives in his little world where his friends are SpongeBob and Angry Birds." She laughed.

"It is funny, but maybe you should try and reduce the hours he spends playing games and watching TV?" I tried to sound neutral.

"It's hard. I'm often at work, and my mother lets him do whatever he wants."

"I understand. Still, I believe a child should be taught to listen to their elders."

"You still don't know Peter, do you?" She laughed again.

"I thought I knew him, but apparently, I don't. I know it's easy for me to give advice. The reality is that I am in no position to offer advice," I said.

I was aware that my life experiences so far didn't make me qualified to give child-rearing advice. I tried not to mention our trip -- or the way it had ended. I was just happy that we were communicating again.

"It's okay. It's not easy with Peter. I admit, sometimes, I barely know what to do or say to make him listen. My sister is always giving me lots of advice, but she doesn't seem to be able to manage him for more than half an hour. He will come around eventually."

"He is still a little boy," I said.

"Yes, he is. He is my sweet little boy."

We talked a little longer, and then Eliza invited me to visit when the opportunity arose. Even though I found Peter hard to take at times, I was glad and looking forward to seeing them again. I would soon learn that neither of them held grudges very long. This is a great quality.

\*\*\*

As time passed, I had a packed schedule. I found a few days to go to the seaside in the middle of November. Luckily, the temperature was still pleasant, and I enjoyed some time with my friends. Still, the fact that we didn't see each other for more than two months made me feel like I'd lost a bit of my connection with Peter.

One day, we were walking through a pine forest very close to the sea, and I was mainly talking with Eliza. She was telling me how hard her life was now since Peter started school. This was something that not only affected him, but it also caused lots of frustration and arguments at home.

"He is still too young to take school seriously," she confessed. "I should have listened to the school's advice. When they did the assessment for the enrollment, they suggested waiting another year."

"I didn't know they told you that."

"Yes, they did, but I thought they were wrong. Peter is not stupid. In his little head, he is still a baby. He wants to play all day long, and he still doesn't understand the purpose or reasons for him to attend school."

"He will come around." I tried to sound understanding.

"I don't know. I was the same when I was his age. Nowadays, the first grade seems harder than it was when I was growing up," she said and looked towards the sea. I could see she was more anxious about school than she was letting on to me.

"I am sure he will be fine. Just like his mom, one day, he will start taking school seriously." I gave her hand a gentle squeeze.

"I hope so. Still, it is so hard trying to do homework with him. I feel as if I'm forcing him to do a terrible thing just by mentioning that it is time to study. We both feel stressed out even before we start learning for school."

"Just give it some time, and it will become easier. Don't stress too much." I really thought it wasn't such a big deal. He wasn't even seven. Of course he preferred to play instead of learn.

The atmosphere lightened when we found a meadow and took out a ball to play with. Fun times returned. I had forgotten my own stressful life. They weren't thinking of school. We ended the day in McDonald's. Peter got his fries, some ice cream, and a new toy from the *Angry Birds* collection. He scarfed the fries down and eagerly went to play in the area outside. Instead of removing and storing his shoes where all the other children did, he put his a few meters away. He also dropped his jacket on the floor some distance away from his shoes. I picked it all up.

"Peter, this is not the place to drop them off," I told him slightly loudly, hoping to be heard. Maybe I was heard, but I felt ignored.

"You should teach him about these things," I told Eliza, not considering how patronizing or condescending I might sound.

"Don't you think I tried?" She sounded offended.

"I'm sorry. I didn't want to be rude," I said, realizing that I was again giving lessons where it wasn't my place.

"It's okay. You aren't the only one who does that. Honestly, sometimes, I feel like giving up on trying to teach him certain things. I don't have the energy." Her tone reassured me that I hadn't overstepped my boundaries.

"I understand. Well, maybe in time, he will listen to you," and I was slowly understanding how she felt. I lost my energy during a three-day trip. She is with him every day.

"Look at him. My little Angry Bird is happy." She had a glowing smile on her face. She was content. It was clear that she loved him unconditionally. He was her world, perfect in all his imperfections.

We finished our coffee in peace while watching Peter play. He was by far the loudest child, the one that entered through the left side of the play area while all the other children used the right one. He didn't listen to his mom saying he wasn't allowed to take his ice cream into the play area. He didn't seem to hear her yelling and telling him to behave. I noticed that he was trying to talk about Nickelodeon with other kids, but they didn't seem interested. Still, this didn't stop Peter from having fun and laughing constantly.

On the way back home, Peter once more was speaking to me as he had previously. He shared all the fun moments from' the playground with so much enthusiasm, with an excitement that I found to be contagious. His smile made his eyes twinkle. This was Peter. He was one hundred percent in whichever emotional state he was in, regardless of being happy, angry, or sad.

The next day was Monday, and I was still enjoying my mini vacation. I promised Eliza I'd go and pick up Peter from school and spend a few hours with him until she finished work. Her mother had a doctor's appointment, so there was no one else to look after him. After the previous night's fun, I thought I'd manage to keep his interest for at least a few hours.

Peter didn't know that I'd be the one picking him up. When I approached the schoolyard, I noticed he was already walking towards home. I was sure from a distance that it was him, due to the distinctive bright colors he was wearing.

Eliza chose to dress him like that so she could spot him from a distance, especially with how he was constantly on the run. His dress sense could, however, be described as awkward. I could also recognize his walking. It was never in a straight line, always wandering left and right. As I got closer, I noticed a shoe he had dropped from his sports bag.

"Hi, Nico! What are you doing here?" he said, surprised but happy. He now had even more long, blond curls, and his face looked red.

"Hi, Peter. I came to pick you up. You will stay with me until your mom finishes work." I gave him a hug, as I was so pleased to see him. He stayed there, shy in my hug.

"Isn't that your shoe?" I pointed to it on the tarmac.

"Where?"

I wasn't sure if he was playing with me or if he really couldn't hear me. He was now just staring at a dog barking.

I went to pick it up and returned to him. He stopped so I could secure it back in his bag along with everything else squashed in there. I noticed he had the other shoe from the pair. I placed the loose shoe inside, zipped the bag, straightened his jacket and his pants that looked like they had been thrown on, and took his hand. For a few steps, he seemed to let me lead, and he was peaceful while we crossed the street. Once we crossed the road, he let go of my hand and started running. The large schoolbag bounced up and down as he ran.

"Peter. Where are you going?" I yelled and started running too.

"Oliver! Hey, Oliver!" he was yelling happily towards a kid in the distance.

"Hey, Peter," he turned around and waved back, not quite with the same enthusiasm.

"Do you want to play? I don't have to go home yet," Peter said as he reached Oliver. I had managed to catch up, but I was out of breath.

"I need to go home and eat. Perhaps after that, I guess I may be able to come out and play," Oliver said, though his tone didn't seem very convincing.

"Okay, I will wait here." He pointed towards the playground immediately to our right. It was a big one, full of lots of different equipment.

"Okay," said Oliver as he turned his back. He didn't seem convincing, but what did I know? It didn't bother me that Peter wanted to play with Oliver. I thought it could make my time easier.

Peter ran towards the swing, dropping his backpack and jacket onto the ground, and he sat down on the swing. I was already familiar with this habit of dropping things carelessly, so I quietly picked his things up and moved closer to him.

"Peter, aren't you hungry?"

"I'm never hungry," he said sharply.

"But you should eat something. You heard Oliver is going to eat now."

"I don't care. I am not hungry," he insisted.

I knew already from Eliza that he will not accept anything to eat until she or his grandmother come home and give him the food that he likes. I thought I was picky with food, but my little friend was far worse.

"How was school?" I asked as I sat on the swing next to his.

"Boring," he said.

"Do you want to play?" I asked, wondering how I was going to entertain him. Eliza had suggested that we come to this park, and it was enough for me to watch him while he would have fun on his own.

"You are old," he said bluntly, though his blue eyes had a glint of amusement in them.

"Let's go over there." I ignored his comment and pointed at the rocking equipment.

"I guess we could until Oliver comes," he said, and he ran towards it.

I managed to entertain him for less than two minutes, and he left me alone rocking. My bottom hit the ground when he jumped off and ran towards a climbing frame. From the climbing frame, he went to the climbing track, and then to the clover, and to the monkey bars, and so on and on.

As I knew already, nothing could keep his interest for long. Still, almost an hour passed, and he seemed a bit exhausted now. I felt great, as during this time, I'd just had to sit and watch him.

After a few more minutes, he came closer to me and took a seat on the bench.

"Where is Oliver?" he asked.

"Probably still eating," I said to comfort him.

"Eating is boring too," he said.

I thought it would be useless to comment. But I tried finding excuses. "Maybe his mother won't let him come outside."

"He's home alone. His parents work late," he said immediately.

"Maybe other kids will come here soon, and you can play with them." I thought I'd found a solution. It was strange that no other kids were there already.

"I think they'll come later, but they will not play with me," he said in a quieter voice.

I could sense his sadness, so I placed my hand around his shoulders and pulled him closer to me.

"I'm sure you have lots of friends. Do you know anyone else that you can ask out?"

"No, I don't have any other friends."

My heart ached when I heard this. "Maybe there aren't many children in this neighborhood?" I tried to find some explanation other than what I knew already.

"There are lots of children. I always try to play with them, but they don't want to play with me. They leave me out."

"And how does that make you feel?"

"Lonely, I guess." His eyes looked like the saddest eyes I had ever seen.

I fought to stop my own eyes from watering. He sniffed and wiped his nose on the back of his jacket. I was too slow in offering him a handkerchief. This was no time to start teaching him manners anyway.

"Come on Peter, don't be sad. I am sure they want to play with you. Maybe you got their message wrong."

"No, I want to play with them, but they think I am strange."

"How do you know that?"

"They told me."

"But you do get invited to parties, so I am sure you have other friends as well as Oliver," I said, remembering that the first day I'd met him, he was going to a birthday party.

"Sometimes, but that happened more often when I was younger."

"Did you enjoy the parties?" I tried to find something to cheer him up.

"Sometimes…" There it was, a little sparkle in his eyes, flickering gently.

"Tell me, what do kids do at these parties? I haven't been to a kids' party in such a long time." I tried to engage him further in this conversation, to help improve his mood.

All this time, his legs were swinging back and forth impatiently under the bench. His eyes often glanced in the direction Oliver went, and his hands were rubbing his eyes or removing the curls being blown into his face by the wind. The more he talked about parties, the more I noticed the happier version of Peter starting to return.

# 9
## I Hate Myself

A cool breeze lifted my hair across my face. Peter was laughing. I heard my phone beeping. I curled the loose strands behind my ear and read the text from Eliza. "Can you stay with him a while longer? I need to go to the school. It seems that Oliver bullied Peter."

"Sure. We are at the park," I replied. I tried to conceal the news. Peter was now zigzagging through all the playground equipment in the park. I felt so sorry for him. Now I was sure that Oliver wouldn't come. I was surprised that even though Oliver did something to him, Peter still wanted to play and considered him his friend.

"Do you ever get bullied?" I asked Peter when he returned next to me. I wanted to know more but wasn't sure if he would tell me.

"Sometimes." His eyes looked down to the ground. I thought I saw a tear forming again in the corner of his eye.

"By whom?" I asked.

He brushed me off, saying, "It doesn't matter."

Maybe he didn't feel he could trust me enough to share the details. It was clear that I needed to change the subject. Maybe he didn't feel he could trust me enough to share the details. "Do you have good grades?"

"Yes, most of the time."

"Are you proud?"

"No."

"Why? You should be proud when you get good grades."

"Because sometimes, I get lower ones."

"Do you think you are smart?"

"I don't know."

"I think you are smart."

"I think I am stupid," he said firmly, and he moved away.

I was shocked. "Why do you think that?" I raised my voice. I was stupefied. I signaled for him to come back next to me, and he listened.

"I don't know. I guess because everyone at school tells me that."

"You are not stupid, Peter. I think you are smart. Your mother thinks that too."

He was silent.

"Do you believe me?"

"'K," he said. He did not sound convinced in the slightest.

I decided to try something else. "Do you think you are handsome?"

"No. Most of the time, I think I am ugly."

"Why do you think that?"

"Because everyone tells me that."

Come on! Who was torturing this little fellow, and why?

"Do *you* think you are ugly?"

"I don't know."

I took my phone out and tried to take a selfie with the two of us. After several attempts, I managed to get his face in the picture. A sad but pretty Peter was captured on my screen.

"Look at yourself, Peter. You have beautiful blue eyes, long eyelashes, nice blond curls, and perfectly shaped cheeks. I wish I could look like you."

He looked at the picture, but he remained quiet.

"Is there something you dislike about yourself?" I continued my little interrogation but only for two reasons. First, because until now, I'd never had the chance to talk so much with him. Secondly, because I wanted to find out as much as possible, so maybe I might be able to understand and, hopefully, help somehow.

"Sometimes, I think I behave badly."

I knew that about him but wasn't sure he was aware of it.

"At school?"

"Everywhere."

"What is it that you do when you don't behave?"

"I don't know, but my teacher is always telling me that, and I know that I make my mom angry all the time. I make you angry too, don't I?"

I refrained from confirming this. It wouldn't help. "You do know that your mom loves you, right?"

"Yeah, I guess."

"Why do you think she gets angry at you?"

"Because I'm often bad."

"How so?"

"She gets angry when I don't want to do my homework, when I don't eat, when I don't want to go to sleep. Every day. But I think she is more bothered by my attitude."

"Why do you do those things that make her angry?"

"I don't know. It depends on my mood. When my day is awful, I get grumpy. I yell. I want to play on my games all day long. I don't do what she asks me to do. I don't like to eat what she gives me."

"What does it take to make your day awful? You are only a kid. A cute, handsome, and sometimes angry little kid." I said my thoughts out loud in the hope of a better effect on him.

"I don't know. I hate myself. I hate my life!"

I edged back, my body stiffened. I barely comprehended his words when I saw him running towards Eliza. I was so preoccupied in our conversation that I didn't look around and hadn't noticed that she had arrived.

"Mommy!" he said happily as he jumped into her arms.

*'How was that the same kid saying awful words just a second earlier?'* I wondered.

"Where is my little boy that I love so much?" she hugged him tightly and gave him kisses.

He seemed happy again. I was still deep in thought and under the influence of his last few words. I tried to stay straight, squared my shoulders, and looked them up and down. They seemed genuinely happy, despite the events of today. Maybe Peter wasn't even aware of what his words meant.

\*\*\*

I went home later that day and didn't have a chance to talk with Eliza about my discussion with Peter. I was sure she knew more than I'd managed to find out. I felt sorry for both of them. I knew Eliza faced similar situations at work, not on the level of Peter's problems, but she told me that she feels her colleagues are not accepting of her. They thought she was strange. They made comments about her being a single mother and about the way she dressed. They said that she was too active and that she had too much energy, etc. I was surprised when she told me. I thought everything was due to her low self-confidence.

I thought the bigger issue was the problems Peter had told me about. Eliza confessed later on that she found out that many kids from Peter's class were bullying him, verbally and physically. The parents of his classmates forbid them to play with Peter. Thus, he wasn't invited to any of their birthday parties anymore. On top of that, the teacher was not supportive either. On the contrary, whenever someone disturbed the class, or any time there was a fight among boys, she always accused Peter first. Most of the times, he had nothing to do with it, but kids copy what the adults in their lives do.

Teachers have an immense influence over their students. They educate, and unfortunately, Peter's teacher was not doing a good job with this class. How did Eliza know? It was the school pedagogue that seemed to be doing her job professionally, often intervening with the teacher and the school principal, always taking Peter's side. She seemed to be the only one who understood Peter's nature and that saw in him more than just a hyperactive boy with low concentration. Unfortunately, the pedagogue couldn't influence much. The first grade was only the beginning of Eliza's and Peter's problems.

I felt sad for my friends. I was angry at the teacher for being so unprofessional. I was frustrated at the parents for being so superficial and for having no empathy for others. Kids are active, dynamic, and sometimes they do stupid things. They argue, they fight, they make peace, and life smoothly continues. One child shouldn't be so left out and treated like that just because they are different from the others. Yes, he could be disruptive with his hyperactivity, impulsivity, lack of patience, and not being able to concentrate for a longer time, but he can't change who he is. Do parents understand that?

I needed some time to understand and thought that was because I didn't have my own children. But those that do surely could comprehend easier. What about the teachers? Wasn't it their life choice to teach? By this, it was assumed that they love children, are capable of practicing their profession, are aware of the different personalities and behaviors, and should be trained in handling them. I can understand that, sometimes, school classes could have groups of children that are too large for one person to handle, but there is no need to always pick on one specific child, blaming them for anything and everything that goes wrong. Teachers are supposed to be impartial. They are supposed to ask for help when they can't cope. They are supposed to care for each child's well-being.

"It is hard to manage a class, especially when one child is hyperactive," a friend who happens to be a teacher told me one day.

"I understand that, but what is the solution?" I asked.

"The system should be changed. Either they make smaller groups, or they give us assistants. It exhausts me to look after a whole class when just one child requires most of my attention," she answered.

I understood then that teachers have their problems in the matter, but they do need to play an active role in fixing this. It is hard to fight the system. Still, a teacher should not tell a child in her class things like "You are stupid" and "You are ugly" and "You are good for nothing" and "I don't know what you will become."

These things and many similar things have been said to Peter by his teacher several times. Of course, this has left a mark on him. Sadly, he can't understand why he is like that, so it made it harder for him to believe that he will ever be anything other than a stupid, ugly, good-for-nothing person.

\*\*\*

They say that the three biggest traumas a child can suffer from in his early years which will make a big impact on his future are the following: ignorance, sexual abuse, and physical/psychological abuse. Yes, trauma can be a consequence of bullying, which can later lead not only to a lack of self-confidence, but also to mental-health issues and depression, among other things.

I had to do something. I had to help prevent more damage being done to my little friend. But would I manage to pull it off?

# 10
## Friends for Life

Time moved on. Months passed by. My life continued. My friends' lives went on too, with their own ups and downs. Nature had changed with each season and showed its beauty whenever I got the chance to be closer to it.

But I didn't manage to be closer to my friends every time I wanted to and not always when they needed me. Sometimes, I felt I was not being the best friend to them. The carousel of life took me in, and for some time, I forgot how to take off and make time for things that truly matter. The company I worked for could replace me if I stopped' being capable of bringing results anymore. My friends wouldn't. They needed me. They have told me that so many times. Maybe I doubted them at times, but I was soon convinced through their words and actions that they meant it.

"We are your friends for life," Eliza texted me one day.

Sure, her message seemed out of the blue, but she has said that to me a few times already. She felt that with my presence now and then and my patience in listening to them over phone, I was making a big impact on their life.

Sadly, I was the only person in their life that had the endurance for everything that took place. I was there whenever Eliza felt that her world was crumbling. I was the shoulder for her to cry on when she was weak. I was the one happy to laugh with them and sad whenever something bad happened. To me, they were my real life, the one that mattered. Eliza's struggles seemed bigger than mine. I was too often caught up in the world of being a successful employee. Market share, turnover, double-digit increases, and rankings were normal things in my daily life.

Sure, one needs to work to earn a living. But everyone needs to have a balance. My friends helped me have a balance in life. They helped me appreciate and experience different things. They were who helped me have a better connection with reality. Their reality smoothly intertwined with mine. They helped me dream while my feet were on the ground, to live in the moment but be prepared for the future. I'm sure they weren't aware of their impact on my life. At times, I wasn't either.

"That is so nice to hear; ditto to you," was my answer.

We both knew her reasons, but she didn't know mine, as too often, she was saying, "Where did you get the patience to put up with us for such a long time? I often wonder why you even bother with us when all we bring you is constant stress."

"You know that both of you are dear to me, right?" would be my answer.

"When are you coming by?" was the question I have heard so many times.

"I don't know" was usually my answer, especially lately.

In reality, a few days or, rarely, weeks later, I was already on my way to their place. I was just so busy with work and business trips that I didn't have that much time during that year. I wasn't going there anymore for better weather, closeness of the sea, tranquility, and similar reasons as at the beginning. Surely those mattered too. I stopped checking the weather forecast prior to my visits a long time ago. It wasn't important what time of the year it was. Real friendship overcomes everything. Ours strengthened gradually over time.

***

"Hi, Nico," said a happy Peter when they came to pick me up from the bus station. After we hugged, I looked at him and realized that he had grown a lot since I last saw him. He was now a bit over eight years old, going into 3$^{rd}$ grade. Time really flies. Eliza welcomed me too, and though she'd caught a cold, she seemed to have enough energy.

"Did I tell you that I am playing football now? Mom enrolled me in a club, and this evening, I will have my first practice. I can't wait!" He did his happy dance while speaking those words.

I smiled, and I could see the same reaction from the few people that were close by. His head was covered now with shorter curls that slowly were losing the light blond color and turning into brown, but his eyes were as blue as ever. He was getting prettier as he grew up. He was almost at the height of my shoulders.

"Soon, you will be as tall as me," I told him.

"Of course, I'm a teenager," he said proudly.

Eliza started to laugh. "He keeps saying lately that he is a teenager, and I finally stopped correcting him," she explained.

"It's okay," I said joining them in the laugh.

We got into the car, and on the way to my accommodations, we stopped for a drink. I noticed that Peter was now actually participating in conversations, and not once did he ask for the phone to play a game, as he had in the past. And because Eliza's cold was worse than she pretended it was, and she coughed every time she spoke, I had the opportunity to have a flowing conversation with Peter. He enjoyed listening about whatever had happened in my life, and he explained to me some things that had taken place in his, the good things. A couple of hours full of joy and good moods.

We had also made plans for the next day. I was the one paying attention to the clock, as I was already used to Eliza doing things at the last minute or forgetting about them altogether.

I often made silly jokes about her poor time management, and she was okay with that, since it was simply part of who she was.

They took me to my hotel in time for them to be at the club before football practice.

In the evening, I saw a message from Eliza: "Can we come over and sleep at your place? I'll explain later."

"Sure, come over anytime." I sent her my answer and wondered what had happened.

Twenty minutes later, I heard a knock at my door. Eliza appeared very angry, and her cold seemed to be worse than earlier that day. I knew that she wasn't on good terms with her mother, so I wasn't surprised when she told me that she gave her a hard time again.

Because of her illness, she didn't have the energy to put up with her, so she chose to come to me and have some peace and quiet. I checked her forehead, and she was burning up. I helped her get comfortable in one of the twin beds and covered her with all the blankets. Despite the fever, she was trembling. Peter was quiet and looked concerned. He asked me for the remote control and went to the living room to watch TV. He didn't seem to be upset that I only had a few channels, none of them being what he usually watched.

After I made tea for Eliza and gave her some aspirin, I let her rest and joined Peter in the other room. The apartment that I have rented this time was composed of only two rooms. One was the bedroom, and the other one was a small place that served as a living room and kitchen at the same time. When I booked it, I didn't bother much with the details, so I didn't pay attention to how it didn't have Internet or cable TV. This left Peter without his usual hobbies. For a while, I managed to entertain him by giving him pens and paper. He lay on the floor and drew for a while. It was obvious that he was upset because his mother was sick, though I didn't know how much he was affected because his mother and grandmother had had their fight.

Soon, he got bored of drawing. He stood up from the floor and took a seat by the table. I was washing some dishes.

"Can you come and sit closer to me?" he said.

"Sure, just give me a minute," I answered, a bit surprised but flattered by his request.

"Nico, why don't you come and live here?"

"I can't, Peter. My job is somewhere else," I answered. I was touched by his question. It made me feel like I really meant something to him.

"What do you work?"

"I work in marketing," I answered.

"What does a person in marketing do?"

Oh! I had to take some time to think as I tried to find a simple way to explain it. I was sure that he was too young to understand. Cautiously, I started step by step, explaining about advertising.

"How much does it cost to play an ad on TV?" he asked me immediately.

I told him an approximate figure. At the beginning, I was sure that I wouldn't be able to help him understand, but I was surprised to enjoy a fruitful and rewarding conversation. He didn't have a precise concept of the value of money yet, but it was clear to him that it was about large amounts. He said that having learned the cost per second of advertising on TV, he understood now why adverts for some toys that he loved weren't played any longer.

"Now I also know why they talk so quickly at the end of medicine commercials, but it is so hard to understand what they are saying," he added.

Wow! I was left speechless. He made me laugh, and I was really impressed with his comment. For a child of his age, who seemed until recently to be more interested in playing games, watching children's TV, and playing outside, I really didn't expect to have this kind of adult remark. I didn't think at all that he wasn't smart. I just didn't expect a child to come up with this kind of conclusion.

"Well done, little guy!" was all I could say.

I heard a cough coming from the next room. I went to check if Eliza needed anything, but she seemed to be asleep.

"Will mom feel better soon?" he asked when I returned.

"Yes, she will," I told him, giving him a gentle hug. A hug that seemed thoroughly welcomed.

"I hope so. I know how much I was hurting the last time I was sick," he said with a sad voice.

We had some more conversations until it was time for us to sleep too. This time, Peter didn't complain. He changed into his pajamas and listened to me when I told him to brush his teeth. In a clumsy way, he tried not to make noise. Luckily, Eliza was sound asleep; despite Peter being careful, he made more noise than he would have normally.

"Where will you sleep?" he asked me while getting under the blankets next to Eliza.

"Here, in this bed," I showed him the other bed that was on the other side of the room.

"Come sleep here." He was a dear for suggesting that.

"There isn't enough space for the three of us, Peter," I rationally declined the invitation.

"What is it?" asked Eliza. Our talking seemed to have woken her up.

"Move a little bit towards the wall so that Nico can sleep here too," he told her.

"Peter, there isn't enough space," she said, laughing for the first time all evening.

"There *is* space." He kept pushing his mother towards the wall and showed me the little space that I could barely see next to him in the dim light.

"Okay," I said.

I tried to squeeze myself in their bed. It was the three of us in a one-person-bed. Maybe it was comfortable for Peter, but I'm sure Eliza felt as uncomfortable as I did. But his gesture was so charming that I tried to rest in that position until I knew he was asleep. I rose from their bed, creeping quietly on the floor towards mine.

"Nico, where are you going?" Peter whispered.

"Just to the toilet," I lied.

"Okay, but come back here," he whispered.

I did go to the toilet, but I went to the other bed when I returned. He was asleep, so he didn't notice. Maybe he didn't say much, but with his gesture that evening, he made me feel loved and wanted in his life.

# 11
## Flowers Have Lives Too

The next day was a Saturday, and amazingly, Eliza seemed to have recovered a lot overnight, so we could spend the day the way we initially planned it. They suggested going in the forest and picking wild asparagus. I was thrilled at the idea, as I had never done that before. I did love the taste, though.

After breakfast, which followed a visit to the store to buy something suitable for Peter, we drove for a few minutes and reached our destination. We were all in a happy mood. Peter and I were singing "I Believe I Can Fly," and Eliza was covering her ears, certainly because we were not so pleasant to hear. The beauty of nature was amazing. It being springtime, everything was green, and flowers could be seen everywhere.

"Don't pick it," Peter yelled at me when I wanted to pick a beautiful trumpeter.

"Why not?"

"Because flowers have lives too," he answered immediately.

"Well, it is different than people," I tried to explain to him.

"No, please leave it be," this gentle boy begged of me.

I listened and moved away. I saw what he wanted me to understand, and since then, I haven't picked flowers again. I stop, admire them, enjoy their scent, and let them be.

I looked at Eliza, and she smiled.

"He started with this thing last week, and I stopped picking flowers too," she said.

Despite her smile, I saw that she was not her usual self.

"Are you feeling okay?"

"Physically, I'm fine," she answered.

"What is it? I see something is bothering you. Is it about last night?"

"Yes. There were two things that bothered me yesterday. I went to pick up Peter from football practice, and the coach told me not to bring him anymore because he didn't want him on the team." She paused and told Peter to stay in view. He was walking and running around, and as usual, he wasn't very careful.

"Why did he say that?" I asked.

"I don't want to talk about it. It made me sad, and Peter seemed not to have enjoyed the practices anyway."

"So what is the other reason? Is it the fight you had with your mother?"

"Yes. I can't take it anymore. True, she is helping me with Peter, but I can't have any peace while I'm at home. She's constantly interfering with my life, and I'm so fed up with it," she confessed.

"Why don't you buy your own apartment and move?" I asked, knowing they were in a rental at the time.

"How can I? I'm a single mother. I cover part of the costs for my parents too. I don't think I can afford it."

"I can take a look at your finances and see if there are any ways you could have some space to pay the monthly installment in case you decide to buy an apartment."

"Even if I can afford it, who has the time to search for a new flat?"

"I can look it up for you if you want," I offered.

"Can you do that? I'm too lazy for this kind of thing. I admit I'm nervous too."

I understood that. It was quite a financial obligation, but it would be better to pay the monthly rent and eventually own the place entirely than to pay monthly to someone. This was the way I thought.

Despite the fact that she was afraid of making this big step I felt that it was some kind of a relief. Her mood improved as we approached the place closer to the sea where we could find wild asparagus. She taught me how to spot them. She told me that I can find them near small trees and even in brier patches, as they like to hang out with hemlock, wild mustard, and curly dock. Ticks, too. She also warned me to keep a watchful eye for evil critters. When I discovered my first asparagus, I was so thrilled that I didn't bother heeding her warnings.

"Is that a plant?" Peter asked.

"No," Eliza answered fast, as otherwise, he wouldn't let us pick them.

"Okay then," he said, not quite convinced.

I smiled. Some lies are necessary.

"Will you help us?" I asked Peter. We both wanted him occupied and to keep close to us.

"I'll buy you an ice cream," I tried to bribe him.

"Okay, one ice cream for ten asparagus," he said.

"Deal." We shook hands and continued our search. I was getting better and better at spotting, but I wasn't that good as Eliza, even though she stealthily gave a few of hers to Peter. I knew she didn't want to fool me. It was more to encourage Peter, as he barely found two on his own and seemed like he was going to give up. After we picked enough for our lunch, we decided to go back in the forest, as the sunlight was getting already strong.

Eliza led us through a shortcut. I saw her pick up a strong branch from the ground and check the trampled grass before she stepped on it.

"You look like a proper forest guru," I told her, laughing.

"I'm checking for snakes."

"What?!" My mouth stayed open, my eyes got bigger, and my body stiffened.

"You're kidding, right?" I said, relieved when I saw her smiling.

"I'm not kidding, but you should have seen the precious expression on your face," she said with a big grin, and I still hoped that she was just fooling around.

"I don't believe you. Please don't make jokes like that. I'm afraid of snakes." I know I sounded stressed-out.

"Just follow me, and it will be fine. Don't worry." She tried to calm me down, Peter was smiling, and I was still really freaked out.

Fear and panic seized me, as I imagined snakes near me. I stepped carefully and felt like I could see one hiding in the grass. A shiver went straight up my spine. My breathing became shallow. I found a bigger stone and stepped on it. I looked at the field in front of us, and I still had another twenty steps or so to make through the grass, but I was too afraid to continue. I looked back, and the distance was almost the same. I was trapped.

"Nico, just walk. You'll be fine," Eliza yelled.

"I'm not moving from here," I yelled back.

Peter was already on the other side of the grass. "Come, Nico, I saw no snake," he yelled reassuringly, but I was too panicked.

Two minutes later, he was laughing out loud when Eliza had to carry me over the next twenty steps because it seemed I wouldn't make it otherwise. I felt embarrassed but relieved when we reached the safe ground. The rest of the day, Peter kept mentioning how Eliza carried me. She proved to be surprisingly vigorous despite her fragile appearance and recent illness. But my panic was bigger. Peter's laugh was precious, so I concluded it was all worth it. Lunch was scrambled eggs with wild asparagus — freshly picked — and it was delicious, but I still had to pay my debt: a vanilla ice cream cone for Peter.

\*\*\*

I had to leave the next day, so they went back to their routine as well. It was another great time spent with my best friends. Among all great moments, I learned how to pick wild asparagus, and I had another great escapade in the untamed places by the seaside, even though I didn't defeat my fear of snakes. I was glad that I was able to be there when my friends needed me. I promised myself and to them that I would try to come more often. I didn't realize at the time that I would go above and beyond fulfilling that promise.

"Friends for life," I texted Eliza while on the bus.

"Help me buy an apartment. As soon as possible." Her answer was not what I had expected, but I realized that one weekend away didn't solve the issues with her mother.

"I will. Hang in there," I answered, and the next moment, I was already searching the Web for information to help my friend.

\*\*\*

A notification sound on my phone woke me up in the middle of the night.

"Friends for life" was Eliza's text message.

People enter, stay, and exit our lives for different reasons. My friends' presence enriched my life and made me see sides of me that I had no idea existed. I felt that I had discovered also the reason for my being present in their lives. My role would be to help Eliza believe that the day when her problems will diminish, if not fully go away, will come soon. Would it be possible? I knew I would give my best. The hardest part is on her, but I know she has the power to resist the negativity until she reaches the top. Then, Peter's life will have all the promise for a brighter future.

Optimism led me on. I pictured a moment in time when my friend would live to the fullest without unnecessary worries. With a strong and positive Eliza, then I pictured Peter when he is the happiest. Only then did I manage to fall back asleep and feel that everything will be all right.

# 12
# Is Anything More Important Than Your Health?

A few more months have passed. Things were not bright for any of us. My health was getting really poor, while Eliza's situation with Peter's school was becoming more of a nightmare. Her living conditions at home weren't improving either. During my visits to the seashore, I helped Eliza look for an apartment, assisted her with all the paperwork, and helped her apply for a loan.

Unfortunately, at times, I lacked the energy to do much. My small weekend escapes were not sufficient anymore. My body was giving me signals, and I was ignoring them for too long. Pills didn't prove to be a long-term solution. The more I took, the less effective they were. While I treated one symptom, others would appear.

"You look exhausted" was the first thing Eliza told me when I arrived in her city. I felt drained, and I hoped that the refreshing sea air and time with them would help me overcome whatever it was that had come down on me.

"I'm fine" was my typical answer lately to anyone that noticed my haggard appearance.

"How long are you going to ignore that your health needs more attention?" Eliza asked.

"I'm sure that a few days here will do a miracle," I said with hope.

"I'm not sure anymore," she continued. I could see that she was worried.

"I just need a long night sleep, and tomorrow, I'll be as good as new. I promise," I said--and I actually believed it.

"Okay," she said while driving the car. She took me to my rented apartment, helped me take my luggage upstairs, and she mentioned that she promised Peter that she would take him for a hike. I wasn't feeling like hiking, and the strong sun was a bit too much. This time, I had a flat with a sea view and a terrace. I thought that some afternoon rest would do me good.

After she left, I grabbed my book and laid down in the shadow of the terrace, enjoying the breeze and the view while feeling that my body was thanking me for that. I really liked the place. I made a mental note to book these accommodations for my future visits. *'I will be fine,'* I told myself.

I woke up in the middle of the night. My head was throbbing. I felt sick to my stomach. I knew what it was. It wasn't the first time. It was another terrible migraine. I barely managed to stand up and take out the medicine from my bag. I swallowed the pill, hoping it will work fast, and went back to sleep.

Two hours later, the pain became more severe, so severe that I was nauseated and vomiting uncontrollably on my way to the bathroom. I threw up everything that was in my stomach. Yuck. I wasn't feeling better, though. I was weak and in so much pain that my eyes were watering. I felt helpless. I didn't want to be alone in a time like this, but what could I do? I took my phone to check what time it was.

"Are you okay?" I saw Eliza's text, sent before midnight.

"I have a strong migraine. I feel terrible," I answered. I hoped I hadn't woken her up. I knew she had enough problems of her own and didn't want to bother her with mine.

Lying in bed with a bucket next to me, as I didn't have the energy to get to the bathroom each time the nausea got out of control, I heard a knock. It was 4 a.m., too early for anyone to knock even by mistake. Knock, knock, knock… continued. I stood up and took a long time to reach the door. But I made it.

"I forgot my phone at home. How are you?" Eliza said, rushing in the moment I opened the door.

"Why did you come?" I asked, though I was relieved she was there.

"How long have you been fighting with the migraine?" she asked, concerned.

"I don't know. For too long already."

She sat next to me on the bed, hugged me gently, put my head on her shoulder, and I started crying. I was still in a lot of pain, but I felt comforted by her presence.

After she saw me throw up a few more times, she took on a determined expression. "I'm taking you to the ER," she said.

I didn't fight back. I let her help me get dressed. I had no strength in me anyway. She carried me to the car. Yes, at least I knew she was strong enough to do that, after the snake incident, though I had a feeling that my body felt light as a feather. If only my head wouldn't feel so heavy.

She drove fast. Luckily, there were almost no cars on the road that early in the morning. She knew someone at the emergency room, so I was taken care of immediately and given a shot. They let me rest for a while, and then Eliza took me back to where I was staying.

She must have left when she saw I fell asleep. I woke up at 10 a.m. My head was still feeling a bit fuzzy, but the pain had stopped. The nausea was gone, and my stomach was only giving me signs of hunger.

I was still weak but felt good compared to what I had been through that night.

"Good morning. I'm awake, and I feel good. Thank you for coming to rescue me," I texted to Eliza.

The next moment, my phone was ringing.

"Hi, Nico. How are you feeling?" my little friend asked with concern in his voice.

"I'm much better. It is so nice of you to ask, Peter."

"I think you should lay in bed until we come to you," he said in a serious tone.

"I'm fine," I reassured him.

"My mom said that you didn't look too good and that you suffered the whole night. Rest, Nico. You should listen to me." This made me smile, but he repeated his order.

"Okay, I will," I resigned.

"Good," he said and hung up.

Half an hour later, they were in front of my door. They came with breakfast, coffee, sparkling water, and two pairs of shining, warm, blue eyes that made me feel better simply by looking at them. They were my friends, my joyful blue sparkles.

The next two days of my visit, we took it easy. We had only short walks during the morning and the evening when the temperature was bearable. Peter wasn't always with us, as Eliza knew that I didn't have the required stamina to put up with him. He was sweet in expressing his concern about my health, but the next moment, he would become too energetic for me. I appreciated Eliza's concern too, and especially the time she dedicated to me in the detriment of missing time with her son.

I spent a few hours alone on the terrace. We had plans to see some more flats available for purchase, but I had to let her go see them on her own. I wasn't feeling in shape to go with her. She understood, and we agreed that we will have a walk by the sea later that day. She was closer and closer to getting her own place, and I was happy for her.

"Look! What a cool stone," Peter said.

We were having a drink while he was picking up different pebbles on the beach. He would give me some of them; others, he would keep for himself. There was only an hour left before my departure.

"Look at this one," he said in awe.

"Here is a pizza for you, Nico. I know you'll like it," he said a bit later, and I saw that he had placed some stones on top of a bigger, flat one and made them look like a pizza. He had chosen different types, and either alone or placed together, they represented things like a mother and son, a sandwich, a rock band, hearts, SpongeBob, a football, a ghost, and a pizza. We both laughed at his imagination.

"My son looks like you now," Eliza said, and she smiled.

I smiled too, knowing very well what she meant.

\*\*\*

Back at my hometown, my job, and my regular activities, I was quickly losing my newly gained energy. It was as if the planets were not in my favor. My health was deteriorating again, while the requirements of my job and daily life were increasing to points above my doable level. Something had to be done. But what?

Eliza went on with the acquisition of her own apartment. Peter was nine years old. He was still having problems at school, not only from his schoolmates but also more and more from his teacher. His books were a mess, and his handwriting was mostly illegible, which caused the teacher to always be scolding him. The time necessary for doing his homework was getting longer. Only rarely could he concentrate for very long at school or when studying at home. The only subjects he loved were English and biology. The rest were terrors for him. On top of that, he wasn't thrilled about moving to the new place.

His comfort zone was there in his old room, with the stuff he was surrounded by and very attached to. The more Eliza tried to assure him that he would love the new place more once he adjusted to it, the more Peter got annoyed.

I didn't have much time and energy to help them make it through the transition more easily. I tried my best, at the detriment of my well-being. Eliza was stressed-out, but I couldn't help much. She couldn't help me either. Would it ever get better? For all of us?

Hope did appear soon, though. One evening, I came home from work at a very late hour. I was exhausted. I went on the balcony and looked at the sky. I was searching for answers. As darkness fell, it got really quiet. Under a full moon, I embraced the silence that surrounded me. I felt I could hear my thoughts, clearer and clearer. Something needed to be done about my life — I knew that already. I slowed down my pace of thoughts. Finally, I knew what I was supposed to do.

\*\*\*

"I quit my job!" I phoned Eliza the next evening to let her know the news.

"You did? Good for you."

I heard pure joy in her voice.

"It was the right thing to do and not because I'm a defeatist," I added.

"Yes! I was telling you that you should think more about your health."

"Yes, you were right. My body was giving me too many signals. I couldn't ignore them anymore."

She often said that I should quit my job and take some time for myself, but I hadn't been ready. Until now.

"What are you going to do?" she asked. The excitement in her tone was still there.

"I'm going to come to your city and live there for a while. I have already booked the same place I stayed at last time. This time, it's for a month," I said, finally feeling joyful.

"You did? That is great! When are you coming?" She sounded so happy, and I could hear Peter in the background saying, "Yay!"

"Next week, as soon as I deal with all the details at this end. I will need to bring more stuff with me now."

Courage and optimism led me forward. I knew it was the right thing to do and I also felt like everything was going to be fine.

# 13
## New Beginnings

And there I was, a week later. It was almost the beginning of summer. I was sitting on the terrace, looking at the peaceful sea and breathing in the fresh, salty air. The sun was setting, creating splendid colors in the sky — a mixture of blue, pink, and orange over a shining, dark-blue sea. The gentle breeze flew through my hair, caressing it softly. There, I felt at home. It was exactly where I needed to be.

The school year was going to end soon, bringing Peter his long-awaited summer break. I was spending my time mostly relaxing while they had to put lots of effort in to improve some of the lower grades he'd been getting. It became a pattern now: some weeks, he would get top grades, and others, he would be average at best. His school success was fluctuating. At the start of the year, he would score top grades, and then, they would decrease almost to the worst. A constant cycle of ups and downs.

It wasn't because he wasn't smart enough. He was too lazy when it came to subjects that didn't interest him. And he was too sloppy when it came to handing in his tests. He also lacked the patience to listen during class and to properly do his homework and turn it in on time. Still, with lots of effort from Eliza's side, Peter managed to improve his grades finishing the year again in the top of his class.

My health, on the other side, didn't show fast signs of improving, despite the fact that I was living a stress-free life. Surprisingly, it seemed to be getting worse. After only a few weeks, I ended up with stomach flu. I called Eliza, but she was at work, and she promised to go to the store later that day and bring me some food that I could eat in my situation. I felt drained. I crawled out of bed to get myself a glass of water. I barely managed. I was too weak to do anything else, so I went back to my bed. The hours were passing, and I just wished for Eliza to arrive as soon as possible. It was taking longer than I expected. I wanted to ask the landlords that lived one floor above me, and I was sure they would help, but I was too weak to climb the stairs. I was so tired that I fell asleep.

The sound of the phone woke me up. It was Peter.

"I heard that you are sick," he said.

"Yes, I am," I answered quietly.

"What is hurting you now?"

"I feel nauseated, and I am very weak," I said.

"Do you vomit?"

"Yes, I do. Before falling asleep, I had to run to the bathroom, and I almost threw up on the carpet on the way there." I didn't say it to get his pity. It was more because I knew something like that would make him laugh.

"Nico, why don't you keep the bucket next to your bed?" he asked in an authoritative tone. He didn't laugh at my statement, and he continued talking like that until the end of our conversation.

"Listen. Go now and take the bucket. Did you hear me?"

"Okay. But what if I vomit now on the way to get the bucket?" I still tried to turn it into a joke.

"Then put a bunch of buckets on the way so you won't stain the carpet." No, he wasn't joking.

"I have only one bucket."

"Use some pots and pans."

"Okay," I said obediently and smiled weakly.

"Are you done?" he asked.

"Yes," I lied.

"Good, now go back to bed and stay there."

"I can't lie down all day."

"Stay there. Do not move!" he insisted.

"Is your mom at home?"

"Yes, she is."

"Can you please ask her when she is going to come over here and bring me something to eat?"

"She is also sick like you. She can't come. That is why I called you."

"Oh," I said in despair. Not only was I sorry she had the same symptoms, but also that now, she couldn't go to the store for me.

"Just rest, and you will be fine. When I was sick like that once, I had to rest in bed for three days."

"Oh, I hope it will not last that long."

He didn't say anything, but I heard Eliza saying something in the background.

"Mom is sorry that she can't come to help you."

"It's okay. You take care of her," I told him.

"I will go now to the store and buy some biscuits for her."

"Yeah, I will have to go too."

"You aren't allowed. You need to stay in bed."

"But I'm hungry, Peter."

He paused, probably trying to figure out what to say next. "Okay. But listen to me. Do as I say. Walk slowly, really slow. If you feel sick, sit on the ground and don't move until you feel better."

"Okay, I'll do that."

His advice made me laugh, and I felt like I was getting better already after only having this conversation with my little pal.

"Call me when you are back."

"Okay." I hung up, and I wondered when Peter had become so mature. He was sweet and comforting in his concern, and I knew it wasn't easy for him having to take care of his sick mother and to worry for a sick friend at the same time.

I went outside. The store was only 300 meters or so away, but it felt much longer. After a few steps, the fresh air was soothing, but after few more steps, I felt sick. I remembered Peter's advice, so I stopped and took a seat on a close-by bench and waited there until I felt better. I made it to the store, bought a few things, and slowly returned home.

"I'm back home," I told Peter when I returned.

"Good. Now stay there and don't go anywhere."

"I won't." I obliged.

I couldn't believe it! Since I had quit my job, I was only resting and had no stress whatsoever, but I was feeling sick constantly. I later found out that it is a normal reaction of the body to show signs of sickness after being under a lot of pressure for a long period of time. Based on this theory, my poor health, whether I liked it or not, was due to my adrenaline finally slowing down.

\*\*\*

## ADHD: LIFE IS BEAUTIFUL

Now it was the last day of school for Peter. I would rather be spending it with my friends, being happy with them, than feeling sick. Eliza wanted to talk to me, but I wrote to her that I was not feeling well and asked her to bring me some groceries. I laid in bed, trying to rest and hoping that the awful pain would go away. I took a pill, but the pain was still there, and I felt a bit nauseated. Not again! I was just about to switch off my phone so as not to be disturbed if I fall asleep.

At that moment, I saw that Peter was calling me. No matter how sick I was, I couldn't ignore his call. He would keep calling until I answered anyway. Who knows, maybe he would give me some other useful advice.

"Nico! I heard you aren't feeling well. What happened now?"

I described my symptoms to him, and he seemed to empathize with me, as he explained how bad it was when his tummy hurt.

"Clench your teeth; maybe there is nothing." Peter surprised me with this statement.

What did I do? I laughed. I could still feel the pain, but I couldn't stop laughing, and shortly after that, the pain was gone.

\*\*\*

Is health overrated? I don't think so. Is it too often ignored and taken for granted? Unfortunately, yes. Even when we know that, we often start appreciating our health only when we lose it. Luckily for me, and mainly because of Eliza's influence, I have decided to take better care of myself, so I could regain some physical wellness. Still, as it's normal to get the flu or a headache here and there, sometimes we could just simply "clench our teeth," as maybe there is nothing to worry about.

Is true friendship cherished enough? I definitely appreciated my friends even more now. The empathy that they are capable of putting in action, combined with their funny-clumsy-awkward way of showing their concern, is the best medicine for me.

\*\*\*

A few days later, I was at Eliza's place. We were having coffee, and she was filling me in with the events at Peter's school towards the end of the year. She was distressed and facing a crossroads. In moments like this, she always confessed lots of other things that she missed sharing in the past. I was already used to this pattern. Never pleasant, often shocking, and probably hard to speak about when the events took place.

I may have been guilty too of not always having the time for her in the past. Now I was here. *Drip, drip, drip.*

After purchasing the new flat, she'd had a rough time with her mother, who was against them moving out. I could understand that she would feel lonely without her favorite grandson, who was often a constant source of laughs and good feelings. Then, Peter refused to move, as he was attached to the previous place. He didn't have a choice, though. It wasn't a surprise for Eliza to know that he would require some time to get used to the new apartment.

Like Eliza, he wasn't the type of person to easily make changes. Eliza decorated his new room with all the things she knew he loved so that he could adjust more quickly. As he was still eating only cooked meals prepared by his grandmother, he had to go to her daily for lunch and dinner. Eliza wasn't glad that Peter wasn't eating at home, but she was comforted in knowing that Peter got to eat regular meals. With this arrangement, her mother was content, and the issues Eliza's mother had with worrying about not seeing her grandson very often were solved. As their buildings were within short walking distance and there were no roads to cross, Eliza felt safe to let him go by himself twice a day. But there seemed to be dangers other than cars on the road that she became afraid of.

It happened only a few months ago. Peter was still struggling to make and keep friends. He wished so much to have many friends and play with them, but often, they took advantage of his naivety. His childishness and unspoiled mind were much more present in him than others of his age. Whenever he had candy or new toys, he shared them with all the kids, those that he thought were his friends.

Sadly, his buddies never shared anything with him, and until recently, he hadn't realized that they were constantly mocking him. When he was bullied by Oliver a few years ago, he was too young to distinguish between good and bad. But in time, that has changed.

One day, his so-called friends thought it would be fun to rip Peter's clothes, undress him, and beat him. That was the moment when he realized they weren't really his true friends. He was sad and devastated. Hearing this made me really angry. I was shocked. How could they? At least Peter finally became aware of their real feelings about him.

They were only playing with him for their own fun on his account. He then stopped interacting with them.

"He didn't want to tell me what happened," Eliza explained. "He came home that day after having lunch at my mother's. His clothes were ripped, and he looked terrible. I asked him what happened, and he didn't want to tell me a thing."

She paused, and her eyes were suddenly full of tears. "He told me about it only a few days later when one of the kids was inviting him to come to play with them, and Peter told him that he would not go because they weren't his friends. I think he wouldn't have told me if I hadn't heard part of their conversation. He was so ashamed."

"That is terrible, but I'm glad that Peter finally realized." I don't think I could have found the right words to comfort her. Despite the fact that it was now history, I could still see how much it hurt her. These events made her more attached to Peter, made her want to protect him even more. She felt that he would be truly safe and away from disappointments only when he was at her side. She understood him. Nobody else seemed to do that. Like any mother, she only wanted her son to be healthy and happy. But in cases like theirs, this required extra effort, and they had to be constantly on guard.

"I found out who those kids were, and I went to their houses to talk to their parents. All of them told me that whatever had happened, they were sure that my son was guilty. They said that Peter was a wild child. Can you imagine?"

To some adults, he may appear a bit too hyperactive and childish for his age, but he couldn't be blamed for that.

"Can you imagine?" she repeated. "Four kids beat him up, and it was Peter's fault somehow?"

Peter had definitively learned a tough lesson. Let's say that those children don't know much, and their actions can be easily forgotten and forgiven. However, the parents could easily talk it over and explain why their behavior wasn't acceptable. But from what she had told me, the parents of those four children didn't even bother.

Not only did they blame Peter, but they were also rude to Eliza. All of them closed their door in her face. I felt anger growing in me, combined with feeling sorry for Eliza and Peter. No matter how strong she was, things like this can easily rip your heart and soften your resolve. How I wished to be able to protect them from all of this pain.

"Why didn't you say anything to me?"

"Why should I bother you with it? You had your own worries," she said, looking in the distance.

"I know, but I could have at least listened to you," I said.

"You are here now. This means a lot to us."

At that moment, Peter arrived at home.

"Look, Mom, I found a little turtle," the little guy said, excitedly showing off the little creature in his hand.

"Where did you find it?" she asked, surprised, and I noticed how her face was getting less tense.

"On my way from grandma's. I saw it behind a big stone. I don't know what it was doing there," he explained, barely breathing from the running and his excitement. His appearance was always funny when he was full of energy and thrilled about something while his clothes were sloppy. But he was sweet.

They placed the turtle on the balcony on a piece of cardboard. Eliza gave it some water and salad leaves. The turtle was slow, barely moving. They usually are like that, but this one seemed scared. We agreed to leave it alone for a while. Eliza kept wondering what they should do with it. Should they keep it?

After a short time, Peter went outside to play with his ball. He agreed to stay close to the building so his mother wouldn't have to worry.

Having been left alone again, we continued talking.
*Drip, drip, drip.*

# 14
## ADHD or Bad Behavior?

When the school year ended, Eliza was called to a meeting at the principal's office. She was told that Peter was a special child, but the teacher was complaining that she doesn't have the time and energy to pay enough attention to him. Her advice was to either move him to another school or use summer break to work on his behavior. The conversation between the two of them went something like this:

"I understand that Peter is special, and I struggle with him too at times, but can't you understand that he isn't like that because he is lacking in education for appropriate behavior?" Eliza asked the principal.

"Oh, I believe he does. He is always saying that he hates school. That is not proper conduct," the principal answered.

Eliza was fighting to keep her anger contained. "He is only a child. Isn't that something normal to hear a kid say?"

"No, it is not. Besides, he is always disturbing the class," the principal continued.

"Yes, I'm aware of that. I was informed, so I asked my son to behave. Still, I don't think the teacher should punish him each time he doesn't sit still. He is a child," Eliza said in her son's defense.

"Look. I expected you to defend him. But it is my job to make sure that other students don't suffer because of one rowdy kid."

"Are you saying that Peter is the only one showing signs of hyperactivity?"

"Yes."

"What about each time he was bullied by other kids? Was that normal behavior from the other children?" Eliza asked.

"I'm sure Peter provoked them."

"I know that in certain situations, it may have been Peter's fault. I'm not trying to deny it. But when the teacher is always criticizing him, saying in front of the whole class that he is ugly and stupid, is that again Peter's fault? How do you think my son feels when he hears that? Is that a normal behavior from the teacher? Is this what a teacher should be doing? Did you ask the teacher to work on 'proper conduct' during the summer break too?"

The principal said nothing for a few minutes.

Finally, she said, "The discussion should end here. I don't have time for this anymore," showing Eliza the door, but the discussion couldn't end like that. Not by a long shot.

"That's it? I have a summer to correct whatever is that Peter seems to bother everyone with, and you're going to do nothing? What about my request to move him to another class? Could you at least give him a chance with another teacher? Why don't I hear any such complaints from his English teacher? Do you think that, miraculously, Peter is showing proper behavior only in her class, or that there may be a difference in the teacher's professionalism in your school?"

"You are going too far here. Just go home and teach your child to behave," the principal snapped.

That made Eliza even angrier. "Too far? Or maybe I am right? Isn't the school supposed to take care of the well-being of a child? Why don't you ever want to take into consideration any of my suggestions? Is this school's policy based on only pointing fingers to blame?" Eliza continued.

"Look, Miss. I think we are finished with this discussion. It's no wonder why Peter is like this."

It was Eliza's turn to snap. "Who is going too far now?"

"Where is the boy's father? I really want to know. Why doesn't he ever come here?" the principal asked.

"Don't change the subject. Tell me, please, are you going to consider moving Peter to another class?"

"No! You know very well that your request was denied."

"Yes, I know. But I was never told the reason. What other choice do I have? Peter has changed a lot since he started school. It's not only the responsibilities related to school have that affected him. It's the environment that did that too. He is not the same person anymore. He suffers, and it breaks my heart. I need to do something to put a stop to this situation. I'm his mother, and I can't allow things to continue like this," said Eliza.

"Then move him to another school," was the principal's cold answer.

"I'm a single mother, and I do not have the money or the time to take him to another school. I'm sorry that you don't want to help me find a solution here. Aren't you a mother too?" Eliza was breaking.

"I need to make sure I'm taking care of my pupil's well-being. I see no other solution than the one I have mentioned to you. You can either work on his conduct during the summer or move him to another school. I will not tolerate this kind of behavior any longer in my school."

"I am repeating. I'm aware that my son is special. He is always fidgeting or squirming in his seat. It is hard to make him stop getting up and down, climbing, jumping, or running, most of the time. He is in constant motion. He may talk excessively at times and can have issues waiting for his turn. I get that. But he is a good child. He has a good heart. He is generous and kind. He is polite now. He never starts fights, and sometimes, he is only defending himself. Is it his fault that his good qualities are not perceived at all too?"

"Did you ever think he may have ADHD — Attention Deficit Hyperactivity Disorder?" Eliza continued, as the principal was silent.

The principal finally spoke. "Do you have any proof of that?" The principal finally spoke.

"I can bring you the proof if that is what you need."

"Without that proof, your child is just badly behaved. This is our opinion."

"If I bring a paper that states that, then will you do things differently?"

"In that case, we can enroll him in a special class."

"Well, why didn't you mention that during all this time?"

"Because I was and I'm still convinced that your son only lacks proper education from home."

"Goodbye," said Eliza, slamming the door behind her.

She couldn't take it anymore. She had to leave the place where she was only met with constant disapproval over her parenting skills and critiques on Peter's account over and over again. She felt a mix of shame, guilt, and anger, along with depression and hopelessness. I could read that on her face while she relived the incident.

"That is awful," I said when she finished.

Her eyes welled up with tears. She took a tissue and wiped them off.

"Are you going to have him tested for ADHD?" I asked. I have mentioned her a few times in the past, but she was always postponing it. Was she afraid of the obvious?

"I don't know, but I need to find a solution." Her thoughts took her slightly away in a stream of temporary mindlessness. I was quiet too. My mind was full of words, yet none came out. She snapped out of her absorbed-into-her-thoughts moment when Peter came in. He returned from the playground, this time, holding two turtles in his little hands. We both started laughing.

"I found another two. I saw the bigger one and assumed this must be the mother, because it's a bit smaller than the first one. The biggest one is definitely the father," he paused to catch his breath, "and then I saw the little one. This one is definitely their son."

Eliza tried to hide her tears. Soon after, she couldn't stop wondering, *'How come these turtles have suddenly appeared now?'* They lived in a part of the city where it wasn't common to see turtles. At that moment, I was wondering how Peter feels about not seeing his father on a regular basis, and the thought brought additional sadness in my already-grieving heart.

I pushed the sadness away and joined them in accommodating the turtles to their temporary shelter. They put them all together; only, this time they decided it was better to place them in a bigger container, one used for plants, as the little creatures were a terrestrial species. They agreed to decide later what to do with them.

"I'll go out again, Mom. Maybe they have a daughter too. She surely shouldn't be left alone."

Eliza smiled, happily seeing that her son had such a good heart and a genuine love for animals. "Be careful, Peter."

I knew now that her warning wasn't only related to cars or similar dangers but also warned him against other kids in the neighborhood.

"Will you help me?" she asked me.

"Of course I will; you know that. Just tell me: what do you need me to do?" I asked, more determined than ever.

"I need a good doctor for Peter. I want to know if he has ADHD or not." She was decided now.

"Sure. I'll go into action immediately."

She seemed to feel a bit better listening to my answer, but then she frowned. "Make sure you search for one from another city. In this small city, everyone will find out and start gossiping about it, and they already have enough to talk about," she said. I nodded.

"Thank you, Nico. I feel blessed to have you here and helping me. I have no one else. Nobody understands me. Everyone thinks it is my fault that Peter is like this. Everyone is judging us and laughing at our account. Something needs to change otherwise I don't know how our life will be."

She didn't need to thank me. She was my friend. She and Peter both were. I was in-between jobs and was enjoying the freedom of doing whatever I wanted, and helping my friends was something I'd do with the utmost dedication.

By the time I was ready to go home and get into action, Peter had returned. And guess what? He did find another small turtle, the presumably missing daughter. He was so sweet. No wonder he got under my skin so quickly.

***

This time, her confession affected me tremendously, and I was driven to do my best to be the greatest support. I was aware that a small town could cause the unpleasant, nosy people to gossip, so I didn't tell her that she shouldn't bother with what people thought or said about him. She had too much going on, and working on her self-confidence couldn't be a part of her plan right now. Peter's well-being was her main focus.

"When he is happy, there is no one happier than him, and when he is sad, there is no one sadder," Eliza told me once about Peter.

I wanted now more than ever to see him always being the happiest person in the room. Was I hoping for too much? While my friends had to take care of their new pets, the family of terrestrial turtles, I was on my new mission.

***

I'm not a morning person. I hate alarms. With no real obligations lately, I was enjoying the luxury of sleeping as late as I wanted. This morning was different, though. I stood up from the bed at a time of day when roosters wouldn't even think about getting up. I didn't have a long night's worth of sleep, but I felt energetic and fresh. The coffee that I loved so much was no longer a necessity to help me start the day. The sun was shining, seeming to send me positive vibes as a sign that things were going to take a good turn. I took my laptop and went on the Internet. I needed to make sure I fully understood the characteristics of ADHD in children.

I typed "ADHD" into a search engine and hit Enter. I was overwhelmed with the amount of information. There were over 75 million results for my search. It would be impossible to check them all. I chose to check the content from sites of recognized organizations and institutions, and I was very soon enlightened.

The more I browsed, the more I saw the same common characteristics that indicate ADHD in children. The criteria for diagnosis in children are defined according to certain areas of difficulty, such as signs of attention deficit, hyperactivity, and impulsiveness.

The clinician determines the diagnosis, but there are several people involved in recognizing the first signals. The main role is played by the parents, the child's school, and other caregivers that should be able to assess the child's behavior.

Doctors usually diagnose ADHD in children after a child has shown six or more symptoms of inattention or hyperactivity on a regular basis for more than six months. After that, the clinician may conclude that the child shows predominant signs under the three categories: inattentive, hyperactive, and impulsive.

# 15
## What is ADHD?

I think a short clarification is needed here, as I still meet people that don't know about ADHD or think that it is used as an excuse for kids lacking proper education or etiquette.

Below is an excerpt from The U.S. National Institute of Mental Health (NIMH), the lead federal agency for research on mental disorders:

"Attention-deficit/hyperactivity disorder (ADHD) is a brain disorder marked by an ongoing pattern of inattention and/or hyperactivity-impulsivity that interferes with functioning or development.

Inattention means a person wanders off task, lacks persistence, has difficulty sustaining focus, and is disorganized; and these problems are not due to defiance or lack of comprehension.

Hyperactivity means a person seems to move about constantly, including in situations in which it is not appropriate; or excessively fidgets, taps, or talks. In adults, it may be extreme restlessness or wearing others out with constant activity.

Impulsivity means a person makes hasty actions that occur in the moment without first thinking about them and that may have high potential for harm; or a desire for immediate rewards or inability to delay gratification. An impulsive person may be socially intrusive and excessively interrupt others or make important decisions without considering the long-term consequences.

Inattention and hyperactivity/impulsivity are the key behaviors of ADHD. Some people with ADHD only have problems with one of the behaviors, while others have both inattention and hyperactivity-impulsivity. Most children have the combined type of ADHD."[2]

From everything I have read, there are lots of situations I have witnessed that indicated, one way or another, a very possible conclusion. The ADHD expert would have to confirm, but I was now surer than ever. Here is a list of the symptoms I noticed that corresponded to Peter's behavior over the years:

✔ He often doesn't pay attention to details and staying focused, especially if it relates to a topic that doesn't interest him, such as class lectures, reading, and homework. For the matters that represent an interest to him, such as studying English, riding his bicycle, and video games, he can be brilliant in taking the time to master the details and remember them.

✔ His attention span is somehow related to his focus. Peter can quickly lose focus on many tasks he has started, especially when things get too complicated and require a higher level of concentration.

✔ He makes careless mistakes in a majority of tasks. This is the clumsy part that made me a bit annoyed at first but that I became fond of later on.

---

[2] https://www.nimh.nih.gov/health/topics/attention-deficit-hyperactivity-disorder-adhd/index.shtml

- Often, it seemed to me that he is distant and doesn't listen to the things or conversations happening in his presence, only to realize later on that he was actually aware of everything going on around him. In certain situations, he would be totally absent, but I would say that this is true for everyone. Over the years, he seemed more present in the moment than before, though.
- Like Eliza, he doesn't manage his time properly. Whenever there is a deadline at school, he deals with it at the last second, and sometimes, he can even miss it altogether. On the other hand, he makes sure he is not late for his cousin's birthday party or that he doesn't miss the airing of a cartoon that he likes. I'm not sure, though, if this has anything to do with the amount of interest he has for any specific topic.
- He often loses things needed for tasks or daily life, such as school papers, books, keys, money, and his cell phone. It is very common for Peter to be unable to find something. This brings a smile to my face, as I can recall so many situations when both of my friends were looking for something they have lost, even if they had it in hand only a minute earlier. Oftentimes, they find it, but not always when they need it. His phone, though, doesn't get lost most of the time.
- Peter is easily distracted — by everything, especially when he is doing something that doesn't interest him. There are so many examples for this that I wouldn't know where to start. It happens especially when he is in school or while doing homework. But when there is something that he

truly enjoys, he can focus and concentrate for a really long time.

✔ He fidgets and taps his hands or feet often, or he squirms in his seat. This used to bother me at first, especially when we went to Gardaland and my patience was wearing thin fast. Then, I thought he was just misbehaving. Each time I remember that, I feel bad about myself. At least I have grown and expanded my knowledge and understanding. I've already known for some time now that he simply can't control his need for motion.

✔ He is not able to stay seated or still for a longer period of time. While at home, this isn't an issue, but the main problem for him is at school. Can you imagine how frustrating it would be when your body needs to move, but you are forced to and repeatedly asked to sit still? I can relate to it only through a certain event from my life. I was a passenger on a bus, and I accidentally took the wrong dosage of my anti-motion-sickness pills. Instead of becoming sleepier than normal, it made me restless. I couldn't stay still. I couldn't stop the bus, and it felt awful. I felt angry, frustrated, annoyed, and scared. It felt as if my body needed to be in constant motion. That feeling lasted for almost 24 hours, and it made me exhausted and terrified. I felt I could understand Peter better by remembering that event from my life. I will never again force him to stay still.

✔ He runs about or climbs where it is possible and often inappropriate. I noticed this happening a lot during our walks. He was always climbing on something, usually something that looked dangerous. He never walked straight, always zigzagging. Could it be because he was easily bored? I didn't check the explanation but at least I know it is beyond his control. During our walks, when Peter was jumping around and his long curls were bouncing up and down, Eliza would comment "Look at him. He looks like a little ship bobbing on the ocean," and she would smile. This would make me smile too, and I would enjoy seeing him happy, exploring all the corners that had been left undiscovered for me. Why? Because somehow, one day, somebody told me that the only way to walk is on the straight path. Who knows how much fun I have missed because of that?

✔ Peter seems unable to play or do leisure activities quietly. I know that when he is forced to sit still, he can do it, but if he has the freedom to move, then he will switch positions and occupations really fast.

✔ He seems always "on the go," as if driven by a motor. His body needs constant action, as his brain is sending him this kind of message. So for him, this is totally normal behavior. Eliza used to dress him in vivid colors in order to spot him if she ever missed him in the crowd. Soon, she realized that his voice was a better indication of his location.

✔ He sometimes blurts out an answer before a question has been finished (for instance, he may finish people's sentences for them or he can't wait to speak in conversations). I know he used to do this during the first years of school, especially with answering without being asked. He does sometimes interrupt or talk without pausing, but I find this really sweet, as he has always interesting and funny things to say.

✔   He has difficulty waiting his turn, such as while waiting in line. Gardaland was a good example of that. As a matter of fact, I will always remember that trip as my first encounter with ADHD without having the knowledge of what it is and how it affects the people who have it — and how it affects the people around them. I can remember so many more situations that would confirm that he has issues when it comes to waiting in line. For example, once, we were in a shopping center in an area for children. There was a mini-event taking place where children would throw a ball into a wall full of *Angry Birds* toys. Each one could try throwing three times, but they had to wait in line after each toss. The winner would get one big red bird toy. Peter wanted to win. We cheered for him, but the more he waited in line, the more nervous he got and the worse his aim was. He even failed listening to the instructions because he was so anxious. I remember with sadness the tears that covered his eyes in an instant because he couldn't make it. He was about 6 at the time. Over the years, waiting in queues started to be less of a problem but is still an issue.

✔   Interrupts or intrudes on others (for instance, cuts into conversations/games/ activities or starts using other people's things without permission). The scene at the beach when I was left alone with him, and he was swimming among the water-polo players is a great example of this.

Bing, bang, boom.

## ADHD: LIFE IS BEAUTIFUL

Peter was showing a majority of the signs in all three categories. I could recognize some of them too in Eliza, but as a milder manifestation. Anyway, she was an adult now, and my focus was on Peter. I didn't do my research to put a diagnosis on any of them, but rather, to better understand the situation.

Now that I was more educated on the matter, I could move on. Next thing on my list was to make some phone calls. I phoned Diana, a friend of mine. She happened to be the principal at a middle school. She explained to me that if the child is diagnosed with ADHD, then the parent has the right to sign them up for a different class, one for kids with special needs. There, they would be part of a smaller group where the teacher will be more able to give attention to everyone, and more tolerance for hyperactivity or interruptions is guaranteed.

*'That would be great,'* I thought, but I immediately changed my mind. Diana told me that the kids that are part of this program will learn less; hence, they will have limited choices when they decide to go further with their studies. *'Peter isn't stupid,'* I thought again. He was indeed hyperactive, had a short attention span, and emotionally didn't seem to be at the level of his peers, but he was smart. It wasn't fair for him to not be given the same opportunities for building his future.

"I don't understand why Peter is only now getting tested for ADHD?" said my friend in wonder.

"What do you mean?"

"Teachers are trained and well-informed about it, so they could easily suggest testing for it already from the first grade," she explained.

"It only happened few days ago, when Eliza mentioned it, but the principal will not believe it until she sees an official doctor's confirmation," I told her.

"I do understand that. Until a specialist gives their final conclusion, Peter will not be treated like a kid with ADHD. But from what you have told me, Peter showed all the signs already when he started school. The school could have at least suggested a testing by now, on numerous occasions. In my opinion, it is highly unprofessional for them not to have reacted to this," she continued.

"I agree. Well, this is a small town. Maybe there were no similar cases until now," I said in an attempt to find a plausible explanation.

"It doesn't matter the size. The teachers are trained about it, no matter what city they are going to practice their profession in. While having fewer cases of children with ADHD may lead to a delay in discovering, three years of this is outrageous. And from what you are telling me, they didn't even consider that it may be the case with Peter," she said, raising her voice.

After we exchanged few more words, she recommended a doctor in a city not too far away. I didn't waste any time and made an appointment immediately. I texted Eliza about it. She was at work. That meant I had some time to go further with my research on the Internet. I was disrupted soon by my phone buzzing.

"Hey, girl. How are you?" It was Eva, a good friend from my country. I hadn't talked with her since I'd left my job.

"Hi, Eva! It is so nice hearing from you."

"How are you feeling? How is your health?"

"Much better. Being closer to the sea, I feel healed already," I said with a smile.

"That is great! How much longer are you going to be there?"

"I don't know. 'Til the end of the month for sure."

"You were really brave to leave your job. Enjoy your break to the maximum. You deserve it," she said.

"Well, thank you. Yes, I really needed this."

"I miss you," she said.

"Me too. Listen, why don't you come visit me while I'm still here?"

"That would be awesome. Give me some time, as my boys are on their summer break. My husband is going to take them on a boys' weekend soon, and then I will be free to come see you."

"Sounds great. How are they?"

"They are out of school for the break, so both of them are really thrilled about it."

"Yes, of course. Can I ask you something? Do any of your boys have someone with ADHD or another similar disorder in their class?"

"Yes, the older one has a schoolmate named Adrian with ADHD. Why do you ask?"

I explained to her as succinctly as I could the whole situation with Peter. She was totally on the same page as I was.

"I can't believe this. In my son's class, I never heard a parent or a teacher saying anything against the hyperactive schoolmate. My son is telling me that the other kids notice that the teacher gives Adrian more attention than to others at times. I never got the feeling, though, that he was ever a big distraction."

I knew Eva, and despite the fact that she was my friend, I felt like she was giving me an impartial opinion. "Thank you for this. I want to help Eliza and Peter, so I'm trying to be as informed as possible."

"I totally understand you, Nico. Listen. Why don't you call Alma? Do you remember her?"

"Yes, of course I remember her. Why do you suggest that?" What did she have to do with the matter? We worked together some years ago, and the three of us spent time together, but unfortunately, with all the changes of jobs and locations and a general lack of free time, we weren't in regular contact anymore.

"I think her son has ADHD," Eva explained.

"Oh, really? I didn't know that."

We chit-chatted for a little while longer. The rest had to be told when we next saw each other. Hopefully, that would be soon.

Then, I called Alma. I had been on the phone practically the whole morning, but I was getting closer to the answers I sought. I could feel it.

"Hi, Alma. How have you been?"

"Oh, hello, Nico. What a wonderful surprise. It is nice to hear you." She seemed genuinely happy. I've always loved when her voice got that sparkle.

"Yes indeed. Good thing that with Facebook, we get to see bits and pieces of each other's lives."

"That is true. So where are you now? I know you are constantly traveling."

"I'm at the seaside. I took a break from work for a while."

"That is so cool. I so envy you."

For the next few minutes, we went on with catching up on things that weren't on our social media. She didn't mention anything about her son, and I didn't know how to ask about his ADHD without offending her.

"How old are your kids?"

"Tin is nine, and Robert is seven," she said proudly.

"They are big boys now! My friend from here has a son, Peter, nine years old too. He is really fun to be with, most of the time."

"Do you spend a lot of time with him?"

"Yes. Lately, the two of them have been practically the only people that I spend my time with."

"That's cool."

"I talked with Eva earlier, and she is going to come to visit. You should come too," I said, excited at the prospect.

"That would be awesome, but I don't know if it's feasible. My husband will take Robert fishing for a few days. Tin doesn't want to go, so the whole summer, I will have at least one child to take care of."

"Why don't you bring him too? He can play with Peter, while we girls can have fun on our own." I was getting really thrilled about it. It would be great if I could spend time with her and help Peter make a new friend.

"I'm not sure. You see…" and she paused for a while. "Tin is really specific. I'm not sure you want him in your apartment, and I'm not sure that Peter would like to spend time with him," she said suddenly. The sparkle was gone. All I could feel was a deep sadness now.

"Tin has ADHD, and many adults are unhappy about his presence. Unfortunately, children act like this too," she confessed.

"I appreciate you sharing this with me. Actually, I believe that Peter has ADHD too, and I think that's even more of a reason for you to visit. You and Eliza, my friend, could exchange opinions, and Peter can spend time with Tin. Eva and I will figure out whether to join the adults or the kids," I laughed.

"Oh, really? That sounds great. But wait, what makes you think Peter has ADHD? Has he been tested?"

I explained to her all the details and she seemed to understand everything quite well.

"I'm sure that is ADHD. Honestly, sometimes, I feel blessed that I have another child too. Robert is really well-behaved, calm, and quiet. The opposite of Tin. I love them both, but with Robert, I can close the mouths of anyone that comments or thinks that Tin lacks behavior management. If I were the bad mother some people think I am, then how come I did well with one and did badly with the other?"

"I feel you. Eliza has only one child, but I can see that she suffers just the way you do. I think this little gathering will be good for all of us."

"Yes, I do too. Thank you so much for calling me and for inviting me. I will do my best to visit you." And the sparkle had returned to her voice.

# 16
## What Is Normal?

In the afternoon, Eliza and Peter came to my place. They didn't stay long, because we chose to go to the cinema. As usual, the ten minutes they spent in my apartment were enough to cause a little disorder. After each visit, I needed some time to put everything back into place. It is not that they were careless. No matter how much they tried, they couldn't control themselves. My decorative pillows were everywhere, and the blankets weren't spread flat anymore. Sometimes, Peter would accidentally spill a glass of water or throw the garbage next to the can without cleaning up. The bathroom floor would be covered with tiny splashes each time Peter would wash his hands.

At first, this bothered me. I was asking them to pay attention, Peter especially. I've gotten used to that already, and it's merely made me grin lately. I realized that this is something higher than them, above their control, so I decided to relax and smile at their funny awkwardness. Other things are more important in life, such as unhurt feelings or showing acceptance, than a neat room, aren't they?

We reached the shopping center. The cinema theater was on the top floor. As it was the newest children's movie, the place was packed with kids and their excited buzzing, yelling, humming, and whimpering. That wasn't a problem, though. What seemed to be the issue was that we had to wait in the queue.

There were about six people in front of us, which wouldn't take that long. Peter started to lose patience, but Eliza took him around a bit while I waited in line. When they returned, there were still three more people in front of me.

"Oh, no," I exclaimed.

"What is it?"

"Look at the screen. There are eight seats available and three people in front of us. Chances are that we aren't going to make it," I explained, showing her the screen above that showed the available seats for the movie.

"Quieter, please," she whispered. Too late, though.

"What do you mean we aren't going to make it?" Peter asked immediately. He always surprised me. Most of the time, he seemed lost in his thoughts or whatever he was doing, but it was clear already that he could hear everything around him. He just only reacted to certain things that presented an interest for him. He certainly wanted to see the movie as we'd planned.

"There are only few seats left, and if the people in front of us purchase at least two tickets per group, then there won't be enough seats left," I tried to explain calmly.

"Oh, no!" he yelled. He then started to get impatient. Now there were two people in front and six places left. The tension got stronger. He was staying next to me, but fidgeting. He was holding my hand and squeezing it. His restlessness seemed to be hurting him. I tried to calm him down.

"What's taking so long?" "Why aren't they showing the movie in a bigger theater?" "Oh, no!" "Move, people!" "Nico, are we going to make it?" These were just some of the things that Peter said. He was so agitated that he managed to shut out the noise of the other kids around. Only one person in front of us, and there are four seats left.

"How many seats are left?" Peter asked me. Eliza was looking at the screen and remaining quiet. I knew she was already preparing for Peter's yelling and crying that seemed to almost unavoidable now. I could feel the pressure.

"Shut up, kid," exclaimed the guy behind us. We all turned our heads and looked at him. "This kid is not normal," he added in a serious, superior tone, and that made me so angry that I could literally have punched him in the face. I stand at an average height, and he was much taller than me and quite massive. His arrogant attitude and overall posture expressed a sense of victory. Over whom? A small child? His big hands were playing with his phone while he kept looking at me, obviously proud of what he had just said.

Seriously, I'm not an aggressive person, but his face was begging for my fists. I chose words instead.

"I think it's you that needs to shut up," I said sharply and turned away, not waiting for an answer and not wanting to deal with him any longer. From what I could see, he was in his forties, so he'd lived long enough to have learned and practiced some manners and patience. I noticed Eliza looking away too. I knew she would be really affected by the guy's reaction. I tried to stay calm. I controlled my voice and continued my conversation with Peter as if nothing had happened. I looked up at the screen and checked the current situation regarding the seats.

"Only four seats," I said.

He was silent for a moment, and at first, I was wondering if he'd even heard me.

"Does that mean that we will manage?" His eyes were a bit watery but held a glimpse of hope. I hope he was not affected by the rude guy's comment. He didn't need that on top of his already high stress levels.

"I doubt, Peter. But if two seats are available, then the two of you can go ahead, and I will wait for you outside."

"I want the three of us to go together!" Peter exclaimed.

"The two of you will go," Eliza finally spoke. "You know that I don't always have the patience to watch a movie from the beginning 'til the end in one sitting," she added.

"'K," said Peter.

Then we all turned our heads again, due to the sound of something dropping behind us. It looked as if that guy had dropped his phone, and chances were that it got damaged. I felt a grin forming on my face, thinking that the universe made sure to keep some righteousness in this world after all. Not that I wanted something bad to happen to that guy, but still, I admit that I felt a bit of satisfaction.

That feeling was replaced with a new one when I saw that it was Peter that picked the phone and hand it to him. Being smaller and more agile, he had managed to react faster than the guy. I stared in awe at Peter's gesture. His hand was reaching towards that guy, but his head was almost turned down as if he did something wrong. The man said nothing.

"'Thank you' would be a *normal* thing to say," I said snappily.

## ADHD: LIFE IS BEAUTIFUL

He rolled his eyes and stayed quiet. I noticed the smiles of the people behind him. I admit that this whole situation created a special satisfaction for me, as in the end, it was that guy that appeared silly and not an excited boy who was anxious to see a movie precisely when he wanted to. When I turned my head, I noticed Eliza's face, and she somehow seemed relaxed now.

"Next, please," the lady at the cash register called.

I didn't manage to see the updated situation of available seats on the screen.

"Three tickets please," I said hopefully. Let it be two, at least.

"I'm sorry. We only have three tickets left, but unfortunately, they aren't together," she said apologetically.

"Oh!" I exclaimed and searched for Eliza. I realized that she moved a bit farther away. She wasn't watching me. I knew this moment meant more social pressure for her than for me. First, she didn't have the same patience to wait in line as I did, then the noise and the crowd were usually annoying her, and third, Peter's inevitable reaction in case we couldn't all sit together.

"Peter, do you mind if we don't sit close to each other?"

"Do they have three seats?" he asked.

"Yes, but they are scattered all around the theater."

"'K," came his normal affirmative answer. The moment he saw me paying for the tickets, popcorn, and sodas, his fidgeting state relaxed.

"How many tickets did you buy?" I heard Eliza asking behind me.

"Three. We just won't be sitting next to each other. Is that okay?"

"Yes, that works. Better than no ticket," she said, obviously relieved.

I felt for them. This wasn't easy. If only waiting in line and the risk of not being able to get what they were waiting for represented such a significant stress, I wonder how deeply other, more important events could affect them.

We decided quickly on who would take which seat. Eliza didn't have any preferences. She easily agreed to a variety of things. Peter wanted to be as close to the big screen as possible. His seat was a few rows in front of mine, but I could hear him commenting, laughing, and giggling the whole time during the movie. Before the movie, he was the saddest, angriest, and most restless child, but during the movie, the happiest, silliest, and loudest.

This was Peter. He was happy, and I was happy too. Happy that we got the tickets. Happy to hear him enjoying himself. Like Eliza, Peter had a special capacity of enjoying the moment. He was there, laughing, while only few minutes ago, he was almost about to cry. The span of emotions that he was capable of within a short period of time was amazing. And their intensity was strong. I can imagine it isn't easy to go through life like that. But this is what they are used to, Peter and Eliza. They don't know any other way.

***

Some things are written in our genes, and can't be changed. What is normal for my friends may seem strange or difficult to others, and vice-versa. But that is how this world is. We are all unique individuals. Haven't we spent long enough on this planet to have learned that diversity is a good thing?

They say that when we are born, our path is already decided. It is on us to discover our purpose, our destination, and our inner and outer selves. Let's focus on that and not stand in the way of others. Let's not judge people only based on only what they look like on the outside. They have eyes and ears too, and they can be hurt by our reactions to them, especially if that means rejection, mocking, looking down on them, wagging fingers, and criticism.

There are many types of disorders: mental, communication, neurological, anxiety, autistic, attention deficit, hyperactivity, and the list can go on forever. Someone with one of these disorders has behaviors, feelings, and thoughts that deviate from the so-called norm. In these circumstances, someone who isn't considered "normal" doesn't match up to what the society considers to be the standard. Isn't it enough that these people need to deal with their extra burdens?

Do we evaluate our own behavior? When it comes to that, we usually decide how to act based on our own perception of what's normal. Is that choice of normality imposed by society, or do we thrive to be open-minded and create our own new concepts of what "normal" means? Either way, "normal" means "average" or "standard." Normal, seen through the eye of the beholder, is filtered by the lens of society.

When we reflect what's normal, it is the picture we have created by considering whether the way we think and act is the same as the majority of people, with only slight deviations due to personality and background.

If my friends are not *normal* based on societal norms, then what are they?

In my eyes, Peter and Eliza are nothing but normal. They are on the top of my list when I analyze all the must-have qualities in a person. With only one look into their eyes, I can see that they pour their soul into everything. They are always willing to give a hand. They feel happy when I succeed as if my success is their own. They cry when I'm sad, but at the same time, they try to make me smile. They are good-hearted people, always there to offer a hug when needed. They never hurt me intentionally. They are full of surprises and always offer new experiences. They help me see life from a different perspective.

This is what "normal" means to me, and I hope I am not the only one who thinks so.

# 17
## The Moment of Truth

"Where are we going, Mom?" Peter asked.

Eliza was driving, I was in the front seat next to her, and he was in the back.

"We are going to see a doctor," she explained.

"Who is sick?" he asked.

"No one."

"So why are we going there then?" His question was logical.

I laughed. Eliza was quiet, but I knew her mind was chewing on all sorts of things related to this trip and the doctor's opinion. In reality, she was afraid that the doctor will confirm what she has assumed for a long time now.

"This is not a regular visit. We are going to see a doctor for special kids. She will talk a bit with you to get to know you," I tried to explain to him.

"What do you mean by 'special kids'?" He frowned.

"For kids like you," I said evasively, hoping that he will stop questioning. As a matter of fact, I didn't know exactly how to explain it to him, and I didn't even want to say anything until the doctor gave her opinion to Eliza.

"Why am I special? I'm nowhere near special. I'm just an ordinary kid. Too ordinary. I can't even keep that many friends. If I really was special, then they would all like to play with me." He had no clue where we were going, as we weren't giving him enough information, but his words made sense.

"I meant 'special' in a different way, Peter. The word can have multiple meanings. And don't worry about other kids. It's their loss if they don't want to hang out with you." I knew I didn't sound convincing, but I tried to hide my emotions as I felt the tears forming in my eyes. I knew well enough about his situation with kids from his class and from around the block.

"'K." He sighed and picked up his phone and resumed his game.

Should we have given him more information? Did he understand more about this visit than what he was told? Either way, we were almost there, and soon, the situation would be clearer for all of us.

"How are the turtles?" I said, breaking the silence a few minutes later.

"I took them to Grandma and fed them. A few days later, we took them outside to a place where turtles live. I think they will be happier there. It's good that I found them; otherwise, with their speed, who knows when they would have met each other again." His eyes were sparkling with enthusiasm and compassion.

"You did well, Peter."

"Yeah. I wished I could keep them. I want to have a pet, but I do understand that turtles would suffer in that little space on the balcony."

"You can have a pet in a few years. You need to grow a bit older so you can be able to take care of your pet," Eliza told him.

"How much older do I need to be?"

"Two years, at least," Eliza answered.

## ADHD: LIFE IS BEAUTIFUL

"This means that you will have to wait until you are 11 years old," I said.

"OMG. Really? Are you sure?" He moved forward, his head now between our seats. He was eager to hear the answer. I looked at Eliza, and she nodded.

"Yes, Peter," I answered. "Until then, you can take your time and decide which pet you want, but your mom will have to agree with your choice."

He seemed satisfied, and a big smile illuminated his face. I knew he wanted a little pig, but he loved all animals, including birds and fish, so there were probably other options in his head too.

We reached our destination with twenty minutes to spare. We were all quiet. Eliza finally started talking. She was afraid. Afraid that the doctor would confirm what she had assumed for a long time now. She accepted and loved Peter the way he was. The majority of society didn't. Without official papers, she could still believe that the reasons for his hyperactivity and short attention spans were only related to the fact that he was still a little boy.

Having a paper in hand with a confirmed diagnosis would make everything different. She would be able to get different treatment for Peter at school. Eventually, he would benefit from better teacher-pupil relationships, and hopefully, his status in class would change. Maybe he would not be left out anymore, laughed at, pointed at, and, all in all, rejected.

But what about the rest of the people they came in contact with? Eliza couldn't just wave the paper under everyone's nose, hoping that it will work like a magic wand. People will still look, think, and react to Peter. Many people don't know or don't want to know what ADHD is. People with a lack of tolerance and strong judgmental attitudes will still make sure their opinion will be known. Peter will feel it. Eliza will feel it. They will still feel marginalized. To know or not to know — that was the question.

Suddenly, I saw things the way she did. It was clear now why she had postponed having Peter tested for so long. I only listened, and it seemed that she wasn't asking for my advice anyway. She just needed to put it out of her mind. This should be her decision. I didn't want to force her to do anything. There were a few more minutes left until the appointment. We walked slowly from the parking lot to the doctor's office. Usually, when the three of us would walk together, it would be a very lively image, but now it looked more like we were going to a funeral. I observed Eliza, and I caught her biting the inside of her lips. Understandably, she was nervous. What will her final decision be? Sensitive and strong, Eliza was both. Which side will weigh more in her choice and path now?

While waiting for them, I walked around, racking my brain, counting minutes and seconds, totally unaware of where I was and what I was doing. After a tortuously long hour, I saw them exiting the building. They were both walking quietly with their heads down. I joined them, and it seemed like they didn't even notice me.

"How was it?" I decided to ask him, as I knew that Eliza would need some more time on her own to process everything.

"I don't know," he answered.

"What did you do in there?" I continued, hoping to at least get a hint.

"I was asked many questions, and honestly, I have no idea what it was about."

He didn't seem affected, which was good. In the meantime, we reached the car. Peter picked up his phone immediately and started playing, just like always.

\*\*\*

When we were finally alone, Eliza burst into tears. She managed to control herself only in Peter's presence.

"The doctor told me that after her first minute with Peter, even prior to testing him, she was sure that he was a pure example of ADHD. She told me that I have it too. It only gets milder with age, and it reflects differently between genders."

I didn't say anything. The doctor's opinion only confirmed my thoughts.

"Why do we need to categorize people? Why should we need certain classifications?" she asked.

"I believe that...," and I stopped. Finding an explanation wasn't necessary; her questions were rhetorical. I wrapped her up in my arms and promised her that everything was going to be okay. Her body was shaking. The hug seemed to comfort her.

"When, Nico? When?" she asked. She didn't need to fill in the blanks. I knew what she wanted to ask. She wanted some peace of mind. She wanted to be free of people commenting and making her life miserable. She wanted a better, calmer life for Peter and herself. Was it too much to ask?

I looked into her eyes, trying to come up with something to encourage her. Her eyes were full of hope.

Saying "Soon" to her was all I could come up with, though I was unsure if that was a lie or just a truth that she needed to hear.

\*\*\*

The following day, Eliza told me the details about the tests. The doctor will have to see Peter few more times for her to assess him and determine her final opinion. The next appointment was planned the week after.

I wasn't able to go with them, but I was filled in with the details.

During that time, Eliza seemed to have accepted the diagnosis, and any negative thoughts about the obvious seemed to have blurred. When the results were final, the doctor gave Eliza the official paper that she could bring to the school. She advised regular consultations with a psychologist specialized in the matter and, optionally, meds.

Apparently, children with ADHD are few years behind on their social skills. Eliza felt somehow comforted when told that some of Peter's symptoms will get milder or even disappear by the age of thirteen or fourteen. Her advice was that it is not necessary for Peter to be placed in a different class, with children with special needs, as his IQ coefficient was above the average, and neurologically, he was healthy.

Eliza was relieved. When she found out that people in special classes often have limited choices in pursuing their education, she had become worried. Luckily, the school wouldn't be able to force Eliza to move Peter to the special class without her approval.

The doctor suggested that she could call the school principal to give her professional opinion about Peter. Eliza appreciated the gesture but refused. She saw no good use for that, as she was convinced that the principal would not change her opinion.

"He is intelligent. He has the capability to learn and comprehend, above the average level. He will always fluctuate regarding learning and grades. It was the same with me," she said, calmly but determined.

"I know that means continuous help from my side," she continued, "and I am ready to do what it takes to help build a solid foundation for his future."

\*\*\*

The next two weeks, we focused on the ADHD diagnosis and school-related thoughts and talks. Now, the time had finally come for the three of us to enjoy the summer. We spent many days on the beach and had careless fun for the first time in ages. All of us. This is what we needed, Eliza especially.

With time, Peter got more and more used to my presence. I was enjoying his presence more too, and his hyperactivity and impulsive reactions were less of a bother. There were times when he would do goofy stuff and others when he would have totally serious conversations or reactions.

"This song was playing on our last day of school," he said out of the blue while we were waiting in line to get his favorite fries. There were many kids playing inside the restaurant, having fun, but just above their noise, we could hear the radio.

"Do you miss school?" I teased.

"No way," he answered loudly.

"Which grade are you going to be in the fall?"

"Fifth," he answered.

"There will be some big differences, right?" I looked at the screen with the order numbers, and ours was not ready yet. I was surprised that, this time, Peter wasn't agitated like he usually would be. He took a seat on the bench next to me and continued talking.

"We are going to have different teachers. You probably heard Mom talking about the teacher I had for the first to fourth grade. She didn't like me. But the other kids were crying on the last day. I couldn't understand why. I guess I was the only one she didn't like. Anyway, when the time to say goodbye came, I placed my left hand in my pants pocket and walked towards her. She wanted to kiss my cheeks, and that was weird. I avoided it, and instead, I shook her hand, told her 'Goodbye,' and ran away as fast as I could," he said with a smile. It made me laugh.

"I know I wasn't the best student, but I tried. I did it because I didn't want Mom to be upset. I still don't like school, and I don't think I'll ever like it. I like fries. Where are my fries?" and suddenly, he became impatient, the way I'd known him to do so many times.

Still, it didn't annoy me at all. I had somehow become neutral to the majority of his behaviors, as I knew already that it was something beyond his control.

Eliza returned from the grocery store and joined us at the restaurant table. Looking at Peter enjoying his fries and at Eliza, enjoying the look of her happy son, was a simple and yet emotionally powerful picture. I had grown so fond of them over time, and their happiness was mine too.

"Would you like to go to Gardaland again?" I asked out of the blue.

"Yes," both answered simultaneously. Sparkling eyes, smiling faces. This was what I wanted to see when looking at them every time from that moment on. At that exact moment, the planning started, mixed with some memories from the first trip. I was surprised to see that they remembered the trip in a positive way, while for me, it was something that I have tried so hard to forget. A reason behind my proposal was to make it up to them. I promised myself that I'd be a better companion this time. Gardaland and trips in general are supposed to be fun.

Will this one be?

# 18
## Second Chances

This was our second trip to Gardaland. As usual, I did all the booking. We were all excited, though I knew I couldn't do anything about the long travel time, and the expected long queues for the attractions. I was the only one feeling a little afraid of what could happen. I didn't want the unpleasant things to repeat.

This time, I booked the accommodations in Verona. Peter seemed to be patient on the road. Both of us tried to entertain him as much as possible. We made many stops on the way. Some were to admire the views, others were stops to eat, and the rest were for Peter to play. Like that, he managed to consume his normal physical energy so that sitting in the car wasn't a nuisance.

When we arrived in Verona, we first went to check in at the hotel. It was a tall building, and Peter expressed a wish to have a room on the top floor. I asked as he desired, and we were given the room he wanted. He was thrilled.

Since we had few more hours until bedtime, we decided to go and look around the city. Peter agreed, and his enthusiasm seemed to stay with him for the whole day. The city was lovely. This time, Peter knew he was in another country and that it was normal that he couldn't understand Italian. He did, however, proudly communicate with the waiters and anyone he came in contact with in English. He was thrilled when they answered him back.

Our stops for food and drinks were short, because we knew he would get bored easily. Peter enjoyed the ice cream more than the view of the Juliet's balcony. That was normal. He was too little to understand. The walls beneath the balcony were completely covered by graffiti scribbles and notes from visitors asking for guidance in love. Many of them were attached with chewing gum. That made Peter laugh.

"Mom! You told me that I'm not allowed to do this when my chewing gum loses its taste," he said loudly.

Eliza and I laughed, and I think others would have too if they could have understood our language.

"And you are not. But this place might be an exception, and I'm sure they forbid it here too," she answered between laughs.

He didn't seem to pay attention to her answer, but he took his time trying to read the notes, and he also noticed people were placing their own just then.

"What are they writing?" he asked.

"Love letters," I answered.

"Why?"

"Their notes tell the stories from their past, their problems, and their hopes for the future. They hope that someone will read them and that their love will eventually be reciprocated," I said, unsure how much he could comprehend.

"'K," was his reaction. Fine with me. He was still too young to understand things like that.

"Can I write a letter to Mom then? She is the one I love," he said a minute later.

"That is so sweet of you," I answered, looking at Eliza's happy face.

"Do you love Nico?" Eliza asked him.

"I guess. She is my BFF," he answered shyly, his eyes facing the tarmac.

"And you are mine," I said and gave him a high-five.

"You can write the letter, Peter, but I want to keep it, so there's no need for you to place it here," Eliza said as an answer to his initial question.

"But then, why are the others writing them if the person they are writing to will not be able to read it?"

"I know, right?" was my "easy way out" answer.

"Weird," he said and moved on. That was the sign that that place had lost his interest.

A while later, in our room, Peter was excited for the big bed, and he jumped up and down until Eliza came out of the shower and told him that he wasn't allowed to do that. He listened and laid down.

"Can I sleep in the middle?" he asked, looking at both of us.

"Of course you can," I answered.

"Are you sure?" Eliza asked me.

"Yes."

Peter was excited about the Gardaland visit planned for the next day. He didn't seem to be tired, even after we switched off the lights and talked about a million topics. And there was finally silence. I was tired but felt content with how the day had gone. I hoped the same for the next one.

The sleep came fast, and it felt solid. The only time I woke up during the night was when I felt Peter hugging me, his soft curls touching my face. This gesture, even if unaware from his side, felt beyond any love letter written on the walls under Juliet's balcony.

Our second visit to the amusement park was different — luckily, in a positive way. Peter was still impatient with waiting in line for a certain attraction, but we tried to occupy his attention with different games or discussions while waiting. He seemed to be reacting well to this type of entertainment, which made the waiting a little easier. It was exhausting, but it was worth it.

I wasn't thinking anymore that his impatience had anything to do with his home education. If there anyone gave him a nasty look, I looked back at them sharply, and they turned their heads. This time, Peter had fun, and Eliza was carefree.

In the evening, we were exhausted but happy. We went to bed earlier this time, and except for few giggles and remembering some super funny moments from the park, we all got silent pretty quickly. If I could see in the dark, I am sure I would see the smile on their faces also during sleep. The thought made me satisfied.

Over the next few days, we visited different places, trying to make it interesting for Peter. This was a trip he seemed to actually enjoy, and not even once did he ask when we would be returning home. He didn't care anymore that there were no pigs around like he did the previous time. He was still annoyed by many things and got bored immediately, but I was showing higher tolerance and understanding than at the beginning. He felt accepted just the way he is, and that was what he needed. I'm sure my calmness suited him. On top of that, Peter was now ten years old.

The whole trip, I had this secret fear that the incidents from the first Gardaland trip could repeat themselves. Luckily, they didn't. I looked deeply at my fears caused by the past unpleasant situations, and I realized that there was no need to worry anymore. The three of us knew each other better now, so everything we did together made our vacation pure fun. I did admit to only myself that I was quite exhausted, as it is not easy to spend five days with two hyperactive people, but the happiness and the enjoyment that I felt were stronger than my tiredness.

The rest of the summer, the three of us spent every day together. We were mostly at the beach, swimming, playing different water activities, walking, hiking, and here and there, going on some short trips.

That was a summer I will always remember with a big grin on my face.

\*\*\*

All good things have to end eventually. This is what people say, and eventually, it happened to us too. A new school year started. This could be another year of being the cavalry for Peter and Eliza.

Still, some things did change. The principal was, all of a sudden, nicer towards them. Eliza told me that Peter's previous teacher wasn't teaching anymore, as she changed to do some administrative work at the school. Neither of us felt sorry for her. The principal suggested that Eliza keep Peter in the same class, despite his diagnosis, and they will make sure that he is treated properly.

"Wow. How come the change?" I asked.

"I don't know. I never actually mentioned to her that the diagnosis was confirmed," she said.

"Could it be the doctor?"

"I asked her not to call the school," she answered, still trying to figure out what had actually happened.

"Maybe there is a policy. Maybe the doctor is obliged to inform the school despite the fact that you didn't want her to. Or maybe she felt she had to do something. She was informed with all the details from your side, so she probably couldn't stand back and let Peter get mistreated anymore," I guessed.

"You could be right," she said.

Whatever was the reason, I was happy that the school proved to be less of a burden than expected. Soon, I would find out that Peter started carrying with him a small notebook where the teachers would write for him important things, such as dates for different activities, tests and similar. With the help of that notebook, Eliza knew whatever important thing Peter would mishear or forget to tell her. Homework, on the other hand, was still a bit of a burden. Less though.

***

Despite anything good or bad, my prolonged visit to the seaside came to an end. I tried to enjoy it as much as possible 'til the last day. My friends' schedule didn't allow us to spend time together regularly, but we did take advantage of each time we had the chance to do so. Weekends and vacations were still the best times for us to do whatever we felt would suit us. Sometimes, we would do sleepovers, and we would always remember the nights spent in the hotel in Verona. We became a super trio. Best friends forever.

These were a wonderful two years of my life. They were filled with everything — good, bad, amazing, shocking, but all in all, they hinted at a promising future. I had the chance to experience what I wanted for longer than ever before. Life at the seaside was the first step.

I have rested and charged my batteries. I wrote two novels, started my blog, and learned lots of new things. I had a lot of time to read many of the books on my list. I had time for myself, and more importantly, I had two amazing friends. It was hard to leave them, but I had to do it. Life isn't a fairy tale, no matter how much I'd like to believe that. Still, I felt grateful for having the opportunity to live my dream, discover the inspiration for my writing, let loose my creativity, find peace for my restless soul, and build solid grounds for never-ending friendships.

The last day we spent together was a very emotional one for all of us.

"I'm so sorry you are leaving," Eliza told me often during the last days of my stay.

"Me too, but I know that we will see each other often," I said, trying to keep my eyes from getting watery. Talking about departure for too long made me more emotional than usual. I was sorry for leaving the beautiful place, but I was more worried about leaving them on their own. I knew Eliza was strong, but I wanted to always be there for her.

"Yes, I know," she commented quietly, her thoughts wandering.

I touched her hand to get her attention back. "You can always count on me. I'll always be there for you, no matter which part of the world I am. I promise you," I said confidently.

Her eyes smiled, and soon, her whole face took on a lighter expression.

"Here are some stones for you," said an enthusiastic Peter running towards us. His hair was now short, which made it even easier to notice his big blue eyes and long, curved lashes. His cheeks were pinkish. One of the things we enjoyed doing together was sitting on the pebble beaches, looking at the sea, collecting stones, and letting the wind, the sun, and the sea air work their miracles. Fairy tales aren't real, but these moments felt like one.

"Thank you, Peter. They are lovely," I said and saw him leaving already to search for some more. I wanted him to sit with us, but I knew his body needed action.

I let my eyes follow his movements. He had grown a lot during the past couple of years. He was getting taller and slimmer, with an athletic look. He almost reached my shoulders. He was turning into an intelligent, handsome young boy. For a few more years, he will still show some patterns typical for boys younger than his age. He will always be Eliza's sweet baby, but he will be a grown-up soon.

True, he will always need to be in action, he may lack the willingness to endure at times, he will not always have the patience for certain details, but he will be polite, he will never want to hurt anyone, he will be a good person, a great entertainer, a creative and bright person, a great friend, and one day, I am sure, an amazing father.

Eliza will be happy and finally satisfied.

I don't have the power to predict the future, but I have no reason to expect anything less from Peter and Eliza.

"Call me when you leave tomorrow" were Peter's last words when we had to finally say goodbye.
"We will miss you," said Eliza.
"I will miss you too. I'll call you every day," I said.
We kissed and hugged and tried to hide our tears. We were all a bit clumsy, and it was funny in a strange way. I waved at their car as long as I could see Peter's little hand moving frenetically.

That evening, I was alone again. I went for a walk along the shore, as the sea always soothed me and made me feel a sense of peace. Especially when I was feeling sad. I was grateful for the opportunities I'd had and for the amazing time I spent there. I was grateful for my friends too. I was sorry for not being able to be with them every day any time soon. It felt as if I was abandoning them, even though that wasn't the case and we all knew it. I didn't want to leave my friends alone. But I had to.

I walked for a while, not totally aware of where I was or where I was headed. I sat on a bench and looked at the sky. Looking for answers, for a sign, something. It was a peaceful night, the temperature was pleasant, the sea was still and quiet, the wind was barely present, the sky was clear, and the moon and the stars were shining in all their majesty.

During an especially quiet moment, I saw a shooting star. Its glow filled me with a ray of hope, bringing the light of the promise of a lovely future. My worries went away in the blink of an eye. It told me

## ADHD: LIFE IS BEAUTIFUL

that life is full of beautiful moments, the dreams will come true and all the good things I hope for will happen. For me and for my friends too.

# 19
## True Friendship Never Dies

Time is passing. My friends and I are miles and countries apart, but our friendship is stronger than ever. Whenever I miss them and the time we spent together, I pay them a visit or invite them to my place. When that isn't possible, I pick up the phone and call them.

Sometimes, remembering bits and pieces from the past offers a temporary sense of comfort. As our feelings go both ways, at times, they call me instead, so it is often that my days are brighter because of them. The right friendship can survive all barriers: time, distance, and misconceptions. Ours has so far, and I'm sure it will stay that way.

Past, present, or future communication with them, they all follow the same pattern. Whoever has someone with ADHD close to them will be able to understand better what I'm talking about. If I were to write all of them down, I could write a series of novels — some full of humor, some sad, but always full of heart.

***

"Nico, can you please tell me the password for my Wi-Fi at home? Peter has a friend here, and they want to play an online game," says the text from Eliza.

I answer her in a split second, because she knows I have it and it is certainly not the first time she has asked me that. My answer is fast also because I know that neither of them has a long span of patience.

"Thank you, Nico. I don't know what I would do without you," she writes back. She always admires my organizational skills. She confessed that no matter how much she tries to write it in a safe place, she still can't find the Wi-Fi password whenever she needs it. But she did manage with a few other things.

\*\*\*

<u>Peter: 10 years old and 5 months</u>

My phone is ringing. I'm just about to have dinner, but I see the caller's name: Eliza. I answer, and as I had many times in the past, I hear Peter's voice instead. I sense panic in his voice, and I'm not sure I get everything he says. Despite the fact that he seems to be in a hurry, he doesn't seem to get angry when I ask him to repeat what he said.

"Nico, Nico, my mother is sick. What can I do to help her?" The pain is evident in his voice.

"What is happening? Where is she?" I ask.

"She is here at home with me, and she screams that she is in pain and that she feels like vomiting."

"Was she outside in the sun, or did she eat something that didn't suit her?" I'm aware that he may not know all the details, but I'm trying to get as much information as possible in order to be of help.

"I don't know, Nico. Please tell me what to do."

I can feel his worrying increasing, while I can hear Eliza's lamenting in the background. I start thinking if there is something I could suggest that could be of any help. I know her, and I know that she won't go to the emergency room, but I also know she has a very low pain tolerance level. Knowing that, I try not to panic.

"Tell me what to do," he repeats.

"Do you have bread, butter, and Coca-Cola at home?" I'm aware he wouldn't be able to prepare some tea; otherwise, I'd suggest that. I'm no doctor, but I was sick in the past, and I know that, often, some butter spread on white bread and few sips of Coca-Cola can help.

"Let me check." His voice has relaxed a bit.

I feel sorry that I'm not closer so I can help directly. But my heart fills up with emotions for this little guy who's really trying to help his mummy. As he is not aware of where many things in the apartment are placed, except for those that are directly his or are his favorite snacks, we continue our conversation through video call. I navigate him only to find out that they didn't have both bread and Coca-Cola.

"I'll immediately go to the store to get them," he says with determination.

Knowing that the only things he's ever bought before by himself were ice cream, chewing gum, and lollipops, the following question didn't surprise me: "What kind of bread?"

I tell him, and he repeats it a few times while searching for money.

"How much money do I need?"

I tell him the amount, and he realizes that he only has half of it.

"Look in her wallet."

"No, I won't do that. I want to buy it with my own money."

My emotions are building up, not forgetting that my friend is sick but amazed by this little guy. He doesn't need to tell his mom that he loves her, because with everything he said and did from the moment he'd called, proved it.

"How much money did you say I need?"

I repeat it for him, and he realizes that he has to take some money from his mother anyway. He places the phone near Eliza so I can talk to her while he is at the store, and I hear his rushing steps out of the apartment. During his absence, I try to talk with Eliza, but she is so sick that she can barely speak, so we stop the conversation. In less than ten minutes, my phone is ringing again; this time, I know it is Peter.

"I bought the bread, and I managed to spread the butter. It is the first time that I've done that. She took few bites, and she says she is better, but now she is sick again. Should I give her a drink? Tell me! What do I do?"

The following minutes of our conversation went pretty much the same as before. I give my advice, and he repeats it to his mom, often adding something like, "You have to do this. Take a sip. Listen to Nico. Take a bite. You will feel better." He is also arranging her pillows so she can sit more comfortably.

A few minutes later, and another conversation in a more positive tone starts up: She is feeling better. "You helped me feel better, my son," I hear her saying, and I know he enjoys hearing that. I suggest that we end the conversation and let rest for a bit, as sleep will help her. He agrees, so we hang up.

I feel better knowing that my friend is going to be all right, and I'm impressed by Peter. Oftentimes, he acts and seems immature for his age, but in this specific situation, he acted as a mature person, as someone prepared to do his best to help a loved one. You did well, my little friend.

\*\*\*

Peter: 10 years old and 6 months

"Nico, what is the password for my Gmail?" says the text from Peter. I tell him for what I believe is the fifth time, and I don't get angry. It just makes me smile.

"Tnx," came the answer immediately, and off he goes to do whatever he has planned.

\*\*\*

Peter: 10 years old and 7 months

I spoke with Eliza a few times during the day. She was feeling poorly. She felt weak and irritated. The previous day, an older woman was crossing the line. Eliza had to spend a few hours with this bossy lady who seemed to wish to control her life. But this was not a singular case. One way or another, lots of people have tried to interfere with her life over time. Being polite or keeping her mouth shut is the only way she can manage to avoid verbal conflicts.

But what about her feelings? Everything has a cause and effect. No wonder she is so angry and frustrated. "Why they don't just leave me alone?" she asked rhetorically. I can feel the pain in her voice. "Why do others always think they know better what's best for me? Why do they give me advice when I'm not asking for it?"

It is often that I hear that from her. And I know that in the past, I had given her advice without her asking for it, but hopefully, I was smarter now. I tell her the usual, and I know I'm repeating myself. This is what the majority of people do. Instead of dealing with their own lives, their own problems, they tend to focus on others'. Does this make their problems feel smaller? Maybe. They may not have a solution for their own issues, but they are always smarter than the next person.

The truth is that people can tell when someone is more sensitive, and consciously or not, they take advantage of it. Eliza may have her sensitive moments, but she is not stupid. She can easily realize when someone is building up their ego at her expense. Luckily, she has Peter, and with him by her side, she will recover fast.

"I'm so proud of my son," she tells me when we discuss how he tried to help her feel better when she was sick.

"I'm also very sad for him. We had a discussion the day before yesterday, and he said that he thinks he is ugly and stupid."

"Why does he think that? He is not ugly and not stupid — on the contrary," I answer with determination, and I really mean it.

"The other kids in school told him. They've said it to him many times before, but he seems to be getting more sensitive to this kind of comments," she answers with a concerned voice.

"I'm sorry, Eliza. I know kids can be mean towards each other, and they aren't even aware of the consequences, but hang in there. Peter will soon gain more self-confidence, and he will realize that kids have a tendency to lie."

"I know; it is the same as how adults make me feel sometimes, but except when I am really sensitive, I can do something about it. I hope it will be easier for him than it was for me growing up."

I try to cheer her up, and it partially works. Still, the main person in her life is the one that can make her happy with a snap of the finger. Or this time, by only entering the apartment.

"Mom, I'm home," says Peter's voice in the background, just returning from school. Eliza asks me to wait a moment, so she goes and hugs her son, and I hear her saying nice, welcoming words to him. I also hear that he had gotten some good grades.

"Bravo to Peter," I tell Eliza when we resume our conversation.

"I decided not to bother with the grades. His grades from A to D do not reflect his knowledge but his concentration and mood on the day he is tested."

I totally agree with her. From what I could see, Peter is intelligent, no doubt about it, but when he isn't interested in something and especially when he's facing concentration issues, his grades did and will always fluctuate. I don't see any tragedy in this, and I'm glad to hear that Eliza thinks this way as well.

"Today, we are going to the beach, but before we do that, we need to stop at the store and buy a floating water mat, because I promised him that he will get a new one." I hear Peter's voice behind her. At times, he comments on our conversation; other times, he is singing. Overall, he seems happy today, and I'm glad to hear him like this instead of being the worrying little boy from a month ago.

A few hours later, I receive some photos of the beach through some texts from Eliza, who says, "My son is the happiest on the beach with his new water float! Several times, he came to me and kissed my cheeks and thanked me. I felt embarrassed about what other people thought, but I was happy. I love my son, and I love seeing him happy."

A few seconds later, Peter sends me a picture with him on the water mat and the text "Nico, today is so cool. Usually, Mondays are boring, but this one isn't. Bye."

I look at the pictures, and I feel a big grin forming on my face, and warmth growing in my heart, because I know that they are finally having a carefree, smiling, enjoying moment that they surely deserve.

\*\*\*

<u>Peter: 10 years old and 8 months old</u>

"Nico, what is the password for my YouTube channel?" says the text from Peter.

I tell him, and it makes me smile, not because he and his mother are constantly asking me but also because he has more subscribers to his channel than I do, and he hasn't even published anything yet. He is just very active when commenting and interacting with other people on their channels.

Because I have his passwords and I was put in charge by Eliza to check what he writes, I know everything that happens. I must admit that he impresses me more and more each time I see his comments.

"Tnx" came his answer. And off he goes to comment some more on whatever videos he watches.

***

## Peter: 10 years and 9 months old

We had our usual video call today. We shared some events from during the day and cracked some jokes. Their faces on my phone's screen looked so sweet. I made a slight comment to Peter that he should get a haircut, and Eliza confirmed that she has that planned for the next day. The comment was an innocent one, and visiting the hairdresser could be eventless for a little boy.

Unfortunately, during our video call the next evening, I found out that it didn't go very smoothly. The hairdresser didn't take into consideration the client's wish, a.k.a., in this case, Eliza's explanation about the desired haircut. He only nodded, which confirmed that he understood. It was too late, though, when Eliza noticed that the guy was using the electric shaver instead of the scissors. Peter was left with only few millimeters of hair.

During our conversation, Peter was at his desk, and Eliza showed him with the camera what he looked like. He was quiet and looked very sad. Usually, he would be angry and talking a lot in this kind of situation, but this time, he just had a sad face with an invisible "Whatever" written on his forehead.

"Does he blame you?" I ask.

## ADHD: LIFE IS BEAUTIFUL

"I don't know, but it breaks my heart seeing my son like this, knowing what he is going to face at school for the next few days or weeks or even months, until his hair grows out a bit."

"I know it's not your fault. I know I'm ugly. I'm ugly and stupid," was Peter's answer.

It made me sad and angry all at once. Sad because no one should think like that about themselves. Angry at all the people that made him believe that.

He confessed that the children in his class are telling him daily that he is ugly and stupid, along with other horrible things. How awful. I know kids can be cruel and that they are too small to realize the impact of their words. But I do believe that their parents, the teacher, and adults in general should help to prevent it. Having ADHD brings a higher chance of low self-esteem, so any critique that comes along will just pile on and decrease the little self-appreciation that one may have.

I'm trying to figure out what to say or do to improve their mood, but I think I have nothing in my sleeve. I can only listen. Sometimes, listening helps. Other times, a miracle is needed to improve the damages. The hair will grow, but the trauma will linger for some time.

Tomorrow is another day. I hope it will be a better one for them.

\*\*\*

<u>Peter: 10 years and 10 months old</u>

"Nico, what is the password for my Facebook profile?" says the text from Peter. I tell him, and I remember with a smile how much he wanted to have a profile. He asked every day for one year until I finally gave up. Of course, it was with Eliza's permission and my promise to check and minimize what data will be viewable on his profile. I also instructed him on what he is allowed to post and what he cannot. We both knew he isn't the legal age to own a Facebook profile. He has only few relatives among his friends on the platform. He never posts pictures of himself; he usually just posts photos related to games he plays and videos that he watches. Once, he posted a photo with fries and a red frame in a heart shape around them.

"How can I close my account?" came the next text.

"Why, Peter?"

"It's boring. Only old people are on there, and I'm not interested in seeing pictures of their gardens or whatever food they make." His answer seemed to be written in a serious tone, but I laughed out loud.

"I can do it for you," I answered, and I knew he would prefer that option. It would be easier and faster that way.

"Tnx," came his answer.

And off I went, texting Eliza about the news.

"Great. One less social media platform to check," said her answer.

***

"Nico, can you please tell me the password for my at home? Peter has a new phone," says the text from Eliza.

I answer her immediately, as I know it by heart by now.

"Thank you, Nico."

"You owe me a drink," I answer playfully.

"I think I owe you more than one," says Eliza.

"That's true."

"Mojito or coffee?" she asks.

"Coffee would be a smarter choice, because you know I can't take more than one Mojito," I write, remembering how she had to take care of me when I dared to drink two of the cocktails that I love. That night, the trip that should normally have lasted 10 minutes instead lasted almost two hours.

"Okay then. One cocktail and as many coffees as you want."

"That's a deal," I answer.

"But you have to come here."

"I will be there on Friday," I answer back, and off I go to plan and prepare for another visit to my friends.

"Super. See you then," she says, and she leaves to help Peter set up his new phone. I was on standby already for the other passwords that they will need within a few minutes. I am right, but I was ready.

\*\*\*

<u>Peter: 10 years, 11 months, and 29 days old</u>

My phone is ringing. It's Eliza.

"When are you coming?"

"In two days," I say. I hear her talking from the car. In the background, I can hear the sounds of music and Peter's voice. He is laughing.

"That's great. We can't wait. We were outside. Peter was playing with his scooter. He already knows how to do so many moves. He was just telling me that he can't wait to show them to you. And then we heard that one song on the radio. Peter started singing and imitating you, and he asked me to call you," she says, excited.

"I believe I can fly…" I hear Peter singing.

This is a song that I would sing, and they would both cover their ears, letting me know that my singing sucks. But I still did it. It was fun.

"Nico, Nico, Nico," Peter is yelling to make sure I hear him.

"What is it, Peter?"

"Life is beautiful," he says.

He sounds like he's smiling and in a really playful mood, so I'm not sure if he is making fun of me or not. It doesn't matter, because I know it's true. Life is beautiful indeed.

"Yes, it is, Peter, but you have to say it like you mean it," I say.

"If I say it is will you stop singing?" asks Peter.

"I will."

# 20
## Peter

My name is Peter.

Today is my birthday. I'm a teenager now, because I just turned eleven. Mom says I need to wait two more years to be called a teenager. I guess to her, I'll always be her baby. Doesn't she see that I'm almost as tall as she is?

My mom wanted to buy me a PlayStation as a birthday gift. I reminded her that she promised to get me a pet when I turned eleven. I wasn't sure which one to get. I love pigs the most, but I already knew that wasn't a good idea. We live in a flat, and pigs need a garden and lots of space.

Next on my mind were fish. I think they are kind of boring, though nice to look at. A small snake was an option too, until I heard they must be fed with mice. I decided I don't want a snake. I was still trying to find the best pet for me.

I told my best friend Nico, and she suggested a parrot. A parrot? I was immediately hooked on the idea. Mom agreed, and today, I have not one but two parrots! If there are two of them, then they won't be alone when we aren't at home. I'm an only child, so I know how it feels. I will never let my parrots feel lonely. I named them Lemon and Lime. They are still babies and don't talk yet. They only chirp in their own style. I can't wait to hear them talk. I wonder what word they will pick up first.

I admit that I'm a bit concerned about their well-being. When we brought them home, they seemed kind of scared. Nico tried to assure me that it's a normal thing, but I'm still worried. Lime, the male one, is brave. He already lets me pet him. He landed twice on my finger. Lemon is a bit shy. Maybe she runs away from me because I'm ugly? My mom and Nico told me that that's not true. On second thought, I think Lemon is jealous of me. Who would know what is in her cute little head? Anyway, I love both of my parrots, and I promise to take good care of them. Maybe I'll be a veterinarian when I grow up. I heard they aren't paid well, though. I don't care! I love all animals, birds, and fish.

*I love to play.*

When I was younger, SpongeBob and the Angry Birds were my best friends. Now, I have other best friends — real ones. I was such a baby for thinking that SpongeBob is my friend. LOL. I still watch it though. I loved watching Nickelodeon, and I wanted to work there. My mother told me I was convinced that when I turned eleven, I would work for the TV network. They didn't contact me. I guess they got some other Peter instead by mistake. I noticed that there are too many kids with the same name. So they must have gotten us mixed up. It's okay. I play video games too. I like to play virtual-reality games with my friend Didi and my cousin Lara. I used to hate Cartoon Network, but I was stupid then.

*I adore potato fries.*

## ADHD: LIFE IS BEAUTIFUL

I don't know when I started loving potato fries, but I do know that I'll never stop. I could eat them all day, every day. I'm never hungry, but fries aren't food. Food tastes gross. One day, I posted on Facebook a picture of French fries with a red heart frame. I like them so much. Yes, I had a Facebook profile. I finally convinced my mom to let me have it on my tenth birthday. I didn't use it often, as it seemed kind of boring, so I closed it. I like *Robolox* now. I guess you don't know what *Robolox* is. It's for teenagers. I know I'm bigger now, but I still love doing things that small children love. For example, I still go to McDonald's. I think they are the ones that made me love potato fries. I love their ice cream too. When I hated Cartoon Network, and a toy from a movie played by them was offered as part of a Happy Meal, I stopped going there. Can you imagine? I was so mean to myself. I was stupid. I see that now.

*I love ice cream.*

I used to hate Chinese people, and I have no idea why. OMG! Can you believe how stupid I was? Each time a group of Asian tourists visited my city, I ran to the other side of the street. I even showed them the middle finger sometimes. I hope they didn't see it. One day, Nico asked me why I hated them so much. I didn't know what to answer. I just knew I did. Then, she told me that the Chinese people invented many things, ice cream being one of them. I love ice cream, and I wanted to believe it was the Italians who invented it. Another piece of proof that I was silly. I know now that Chinese people are the same as any other person. I would apologize to all of them for being rude in the past, even if only in my thoughts. But how would I know who they were? They all look so much alike. How do they distinguish themselves? Beats me.

*I love pigs.*
My aunt is a cannibal. The other day I caught her eating, and I asked her what it was. She said it was pork. What? How can she eat pork? Don't get me wrong; I know what a cannibal is. For me, animals are the same as humans. Pigs are also living creatures. They are so sweet. I wish I could have one in my home. I hope my aunt won't eat them all. God, when did you leave us?

*I love candy.*
In all shapes, colors, and flavors. My mom doesn't know it but the only reason I eat my meal at the grandma's is because I get a candy after. Why else would I eat something I don't like? When I'm an adult, I will let my kids eat only what they love. Well, Mom tells me that candy is bad for my teeth. I guess she is right, because some of them turned brown and fell out. Is that why SpongeBob has only two teeth? Did he eat lots of candies?

*I love snow.*
My whole life, it's only snowed twice in my city. I wished it would have snowed all the time during the winter. I want to make a snowman. I made one two years ago when we went to another city. There was so much snow everywhere. Wonderful! Breathing in the chilly air and playing with snow was so much fun. Snowball fights. Snow Angels. Making fresh footsteps in the snow. Jumping from footstep to footstep and

see who can stay in without falling out. It was a blast. I will ask my mom to go again unless it will snow more in my city.

*I hate school.*
I don't know who invented school. I know that if I study, my life will be easier later on and I can get a better job than without school, but this doesn't make me hate it less. I remember that my life was much nicer before I started going to school. Of course, I don't remember everything, but my mother and grandmother are always telling me stories about those times.

I was hilarious. One day, when I was three, I was at a concert with my mom, and I ran off from her arms and went to the stage and grabbed the guitar from the hands of the singer. Mom felt embarrassed; everyone was laughing. I laugh each time my mother tells me that story. I wish I could remember it. I was too little. At three years old — can you imagine how cheeky I was? Due to that special event, I received a small guitar as a present from Nico. I somehow knew how to use it already and started playing it right away. At least, that's what my mom told me.

She exaggerates a lot, though. I know that. She tells me that I'm handsome, but she is biased. I know I'm not, because other people tell me otherwise.

She tells me that I'm smart. I know I'm not, because if I was, then I would love going to school and doing homework. Okay. Sometimes I think I'm a little bit smart. I don't know why, but at times, I get top grades. I can get the highest grade when we do some tests, and other times, I get the worst score.

My mind gets strange when I take a test. I can't always concentrate and remember stuff. I see the birds flying outside the window, the kid in front of me scratching her head, some noise coming from the hallway. Wait, what was I supposed to do? The teacher was asking me a question. What question? Too late.

Maybe I don't hate school. I just don't like it. I love school vacations when I'm not forced to sit in one place, do homework, and memorize the names of all the plants, rivers, mountains, and countries that exist in the world. Who needs to know all that?

I like English class. I'm pretty good at English. I know almost every word, and if there is one I don't understand, I go on the Internet and use Google Translate.

Some time ago, a boy from my class asked the English teacher who her favorite student was. She answered by saying, "Peter." I said, "What?" And she confirmed and smiled. My cheeks turned red. My eyes turned to the floor. I felt embarrassed. I'm not used to being anybody's favorite, except for my mom. Why would she say that?

Maybe she also thinks that my English is good. I talk with Nico and my friend Didi in English often. It felt good after all to know the teacher's opinion of me. I guess other kids didn't like hearing it. I did. I only hope they won't hate me more because of that.

*I love summertime.*

Each time the school year ends, I'm so happy, just the happiest. I was especially happy when I finished 4th grade. The last day of school, all my schoolmates were crying because it was the last day with this teacher. I was the only one that didn't cry. I guess she didn't like me either.

As a matter of fact, I'm quite sure she didn't. On the last day, I said goodbye and immediately turned around and left. The crybabies were still there. I was free, and not only was it finally summer vacation, but I didn't have to see that teacher again. I bet she was glad too, because she always criticized me. I love summer because the temperature feels so good and I get to go to the beach every day.

Now that I'm bigger, I can enjoy more. I can jump or snorkel. When I was a baby, I think I was bored at the beach. The other day, my mother invited her friend Gigi and her toddler to come with us. I love babies. They are so cute and funny. I played with the baby in not-so-deep water, he was happy, and he was laughing. Gigi went to swim while I and Mom watched over the baby.

What fun the three of us had! I didn't have as much time for jumping, but this was fun too. The baby enjoyed it too. I don't know what happened to Gigi, though. When we dropped the two of them off, she told my mom that she doesn't want to see me anymore. I was not a good influence for her baby, she added. Weird. I guess she didn't want me to hear it. But I did, and I was confused. What did I do? Mom told her that, in that case, they won't see each other at all and took off. I could see she was angry. I know people think I am ugly and weird. I think that is why my mother felt like crying that moment.

I think I'm still too small to understand adults. Before we went to sleep, I asked my mom why Gigi had said that. She asked me to forget it. Some people are just too narrow-minded and whoever will not accept me will be out of our lives. I guess I need to wait a few more years before I can understand this. The next day, we went again to the beach, just the two of us. It was fun. I had more time to jump and snorkel. But I need to be careful in the strong sun as it may turn me into a fried chicken.

*I love wintertime too.*
Not only because of the snow as I don't see it often. Mostly because of all the gifts I receive and the holiday spirit. I wish that all the children would receive gifts from Santa. Last Christmas, I wrote to Santa to bring me only a small gift and the rest to give to the poor children. I hope he listened to me.

*I love New York.*
Once, for school, I had to write about something that I wished for. I decided to write about New York City, which didn't surprise anyone. In my story, I was a little boy that found an old fridge and a computer in the attic and decided to build a time machine. Actually, it was going to be a teleporter that would take me directly to Times Square. I managed to make the machine work, but it took me the whole day to build it. I was exhausted. I laid down a bit before pressing the start button. I fell asleep.

One day, I will travel to New York. This is where I want to go when I grow up. Mom and Nico said that we will go together. I can't wait. All other cities look depressing. I only like modern cities. New York is a modern city.

Why would anyone want to live in an old building? What if there are ghosts inside the houses? Not that I'm afraid. I'm not afraid of anything. I'm strong. I can watch horror movies and play scary games. My mom is always afraid of that stuff. When we watch a horror movie together, she gets so scared that I feel sorry for her and turn it off. I'm not afraid. No. She's the only one of us who gets scared. I only stop watching because of her.

*I love technology.*
I'm glad I grew up in a time with the Internet and all the other discoveries in modern technology. My mom told me what her childhood looked like. I think it's fun to go outside, but it is so much fun to play video games, watch YouTube, and watch TV. My latest acquisition that I purchased with my own money — well, the money that my dad gave me the last time he visited me — is a VR[3] headset. I'm so hooked on it. I only have to make sure I don't play it for too long, because it can make my head hurt. I also need to pay attention when I move so I don't run into anything or fall down. But it's so cool. I wish time could pass faster so that technology can advance even more. I can't wait for all the new inventions. I'll be the first one to use the new things.

*I love having friends.*
I guess it's normal to wish I had friends. I remember that I was depressed about a year ago. By that, I mean that I was sad about not having friends. I felt lonely and often got bored playing by myself in the house all day long. I did spent lots of time with my mom and sometimes with relatives or her friends, but not with kids my age. They didn't want to play with me anymore. I don't know why. Maybe they thought I

---
[3] Virtual reality

was ugly. Mom tells me all the time that I look good. But I know this is what moms say. I'm her son, so it's normal for her to think that. Now, I have a few friends. I love spending time with them. I guess they feel the same; otherwise, they wouldn't invite me to do things with them all the time. Next door to my aunt's house lives this girl, Didi. She is a lot younger than me, by almost 5 months. But she is cool. We speak in English and like to play the same games. Sometimes she looks at me funny. I don't know what that means. I guess she likes me. I like her too. She is not boring at all.

*I love to ride my bicycle.*

My trainer thinks I'm talented. I guess I am if he says so. I know that I enjoy riding my bicycle, especially off-road. There are parts of our regular training that are up on the hill. I can deal with it without problems. Other kids, older than me, stop. They say they are afraid. I'm not afraid. I'm the youngest in the group. I was the only one going to the last three competitions in other cities from my country. I even appeared in the news holding the cup. They say I'm the star of the club, and even of the city. I guess there might be some truth in it. All I know is that I love riding my bicycle, and it is never boring, unlike other things, like homework. They also say I'm a fast runner. The fastest. They say I'm a good football player. I guess I am. And now the boys from my class are fighting over me every time we play. They want me to be a part of their team. My mother was a football star. We are a lot alike, so I must have gotten this from her too. My mom is so cool. I couldn't wish for a better one. I love her.

## ADHD: LIFE IS BEAUTIFUL

*I have ADHD.*

Honestly, I have no clue what that is, but the doctor told me I have it. I hear people talking about it every once in a while. I don't know if it's good or bad, but I'm not sure if anyone else has it. Maybe my cousin. I heard my aunt saying something the other day. She was also apologizing to my mom that now she doesn't think anymore that my mom raised me badly, because her son is acting exactly like I do. I love my cousin. He is so cool. I can't wait for him to grow up, so we can have even more things in common. He is too little for now.

But really? What is this "ADHD"? I don't want to ask my mom, because she gets upset whenever she hears someone mention this word. As far as I'm concerned, as long as I don't see it, I don't have it. Maybe it is something like in my VR games.

Maybe ADHD is a kind of superpower that you have to have in order to reach the final level. I guess that's it. I love playing my games. I'm very good at it and Mom is always angry about it. That must be it! I have a superpower. I win! I'm so cool. Yay!

# 21
## Eliza

My name is Eliza.

I was born in a small city by the sea. I've loved running as far back as I can remember. Sometimes, I run for fun, as it's healthy exercise for my well-being, and sometimes, to burn out the anxiety building in me, and sometimes, to escape from people.

My life isn't always easy, but I would be lying if I said it didn't have happy moments. I'm grateful for the good parts, but they don't always last for long. Often, it feels too hard. I walked on the corridor of life not seeing the tiny hope. I trudge off down the hall, dejected and mad at the world, thinking, *'Why is this happening to me? Why me? What have I done wrong?'* In time, I've come to understand that life is teaching me lessons. Lessons that I should have perhaps learned earlier. But it is never too late to start.

There is a favorite spot in the city, at the top of the hill. I love going there and being on my own. The view is splendid. On one side, I see the sea and on the other, the highway. Usually, I admire the sea, but there are moments when I look the other direction.

I watch the traffic go by, and too often, it resembles my life. There are no traffic lights on the highway — only the speed limit and the unexpected maneuvers of the other drivers. Sometimes, they overpass me, and sometimes, I feel I could drive at my own speed without feeling the need to push the brakes. Then I smile, maybe not entirely, as I need to be prepared for the dangers that may come my way. Dangers can surprise me anytime. In critical situations, others may do something that would affect my driving, a.k.a. my life.

Then my halfhearted smile vanishes, and I can see in the mirror a tense frown taking its place. One by one, they all leave marks on my face, on my life. There are many wrinkles on my face, many of them due to worries and sadness.

Will it ever end?

Was I not grateful enough for the good moments, and I'm now being punished?

Is this maybe how life should be? Full of ups and downs, not knowing what will happen next?

Why does it always happen to me? These are questions I ask myself often. The only answer I could find is the same: lessons that I need to learn. Haven't I learned enough at this point?

I know now that it's better late than never, that I can do something about it. It's similar to the cars. With a safer model and a smarter way of driving, I can be out of danger. I love to drive. Not only cars. Now, I love my life like never before. If I thought about all the dangers that may happen on the road, I'd never sit in a car again. But I keep on driving, sometimes at a regular speed, slower or faster at times, depending on what the road requires. I love adrenaline, but I also enjoy the calm moments. Then I can take the time and admire the view. Is it okay to feel calm sometimes? It happens so rarely.

I know I need to rid myself of the burdens of fear, negativity, and self-doubt. I need to put myself solidly on the track toward a brighter future. Recently, I enrolled for university. I know this will require better time management and prioritization, but I believe I can manage it. This is one thing that I've postponed for such a long time, and now, it needs to be done.

Peter is 11 years old now. He still requires a lot of time and patience, but he is changing into a well-behaved teenager. He encourages me to continue my studies. He still doesn't love school, but it is clear to him that better education may lead to a better future — for both of us.

Looking at him now, I can see that I have done a good job. He has changed so much in only a few years. Now, he is extremely polite and waves to everyone, when the situation requires it. He is more conscious regarding school. He isn't excited to do his homework, but he doesn't need to be reminded and yelled at several times before he starts doing it. His schoolbooks still look messy. He still has problems finding things in his backpack and bringing everything back from school. There are still situations when he might not have time to finish an in-class assignment or he has forgotten an important message from the teacher. The other day, he missed out on a field trip because the permission slip got lost in his overflowing backpack.

He may repeatedly get in trouble for having a cluttered room, even after being told to tidy it up. I know now that this is beyond him. His grandmother knows it too. I hope that any other close person in his life will find place in their heart for understanding. He will tidy up his room and think he did a great job, while other people might think that the room is messier than before.

At the end of the day, does that really matter? I'd rather have a clean and happy child than a miserable one in a room that is always in tip-top shape. All these things will probably always manifest in one way or another. The change of the teacher had a big impact on Peter's behavior and general satisfaction. He changed for the better drastically during the past two years. As a consequence, it impacted my life too.

I'm aware Peter will always be a bit different than others, but I'm less worried now. I've been different my whole life too, so if anyone can understand him, it's me. It is not easy going through life constantly being the one that differs so clearly from the rest in the family, at school, at work, among friends. But yet, life can be still amazing, even being someone that stands out as being different. I have learned a lot over the years, and I'll continue working on myself. I'm well aware of what awaits for Peter. But I know I can help him. I will continue doing my best to make him strong for anything bad that could come his way.

There are still things that need to be corrected. He still often says that he is ugly, and I try not to react each time, but it hurts. There is one girl that seems to fancy him, and I count on that to influence his self-perception. He is only 11, but at times, he seems to be a grown-up already. He is the most empathetic and goodhearted person I know.

I was told a few years ago that Peter has ADHD and that I may have it too. What now? I'm not sure how I feel about it even today. I asked myself this: What am I supposed to do?

There were many unknowns, but I know I need to make smart decisions. Even if I'd rather live in denial, I know I need to consider what it's best for Peter. I'm the most important person in his life, and his future depends on me. I did and will do whatever it takes to strengthen myself, to have the power to fight against all the barriers, both seen and unseen. I never asked the doctor to give me the written confirmation. I never used the verbal confirmation of the diagnosis at school or at any gathering.

I realize that I can't prepare the road ahead for Peter to go easier in life, but I can try to prepare him. I'm aware that it would be much easier for Peter, for kids like him, for me and for anyone else that differs from the majority, if there would be more tolerance, greater understanding, and less judgment.

Peter is very similar to me, from all points of view. He is actually a better version of me. I know now that I did some things right after all. I do hope that when people see him now, they may reconsider any older judgments they had regarding hyperactive kids with attention deficit problems. Every person deserves the chance to enjoy the life to the fullest and feel a welcome part of the world they live in. Today, I see things more clearly, though it wasn't always like this.

I think I lost sight of myself in the midst of all the troubles that I faced in my life, on the road. Until a few years ago, I used to be able to feel the happiness and embrace the beauty of life, despite the hard moments. Since Peter started to go to school, because of all the new problems and obligations that appeared, I felt kind of lost in the shuffle. On top of that, ADHD made me weak. It made me feel powerless, inhibited, and guilty. Guilty, because I may have not been the best mother. That I may have not learned how to take better care of my son. That I wasn't brave enough or smart enough to know how to protect him. That I may have failed in offering him a happy childhood. That I should have done things differently already, in order for things to change. For the better.

I know it isn't too late. Now, it's finally time to create a life of fulfillment.

When I look back on these days, I will see things differently than when I lived them. There are days when I forget that life is like a river. It never has peace, and it follows its natural, flowing course. I don't need peace. I like to be the river; I just wish there would be fewer obstacles on the way.

Sometimes, years later, old accidents of fate will bring a positive turnout that wouldn't happen without patience. And then the river that resembles my life will have a wider stream. The rain and the snow were necessary.

In retrospect, I can see that my mother's reaction when she found out I was pregnant had a positive impact on my life. I forgave her. She wanted to teach me a lesson. Sometimes, the best lessons are learned the tougher way. I've certainly learned mine. Despite the hard times she gave me during all these years, I feel a strong sense of gratitude for my mother. She is one of the people that helped me tremendously during the hardest times. As strange as it can sound, she was my rock through my life. I have no doubt that she will continue to be. I'm happy that Peter has such a loving grandmother.

I'm grateful to Peter's father too. We weren't meant to be together, but the best thing possible came out of our short-term relationship: Peter. He is not just my son. He is my baby, my love, my world, my everything.

I'm grateful to the few good people that have crossed my life. Some stayed, and some have left already, but they all left their mark on me. I know there are still good people out there, and I know I'm going to meet new ones on my path. I'm raising my son to be one of them. I can already see that I'm doing a hell of a job.

Without Peter, I feel I wouldn't have grown as a person. I wouldn't have reached so deep within myself. Despite the hard moments, I don't think I would have managed to do that if I had not had him. He keeps me alive. He makes my life complete. He gives my life meaning. I'm not sure I would ever find anything so close, so uplifting, so fulfilling if he hadn't been born. We are bonded for life.

I say to Peter with or without words, today, tomorrow, and forever: "You are my fighter, my winner, my life. The day you were born had changed my world and gave it color and a new meaning. I love you so much, and I hope my love and guidance will keep you safe from all the bad things in the world. Accept the fact that you are different, and be proud of it. Don't change. The right people will know to appreciate you for who you are. Don't worry too much. Live your life. Smile. Be happy. I'll always be by your side."

The landscape near my city is picturesque, and so is my life. The surrounding hills and off-roads are often full of sharp stones. This part of the world has never had dangerous weather like hurricanes. But my life has. I know these storms made me stronger; they helped me see the good side in everything. They forced me to move forward. At the same time, they encouraged me to learn how to take small breaks, to look around, to be thankful for, and content with, what I see and what I have.

Whenever I stop at my favorite spot at the top of the hill, the view over the sea calms me, offering a sight that often says much more than the eyes can see.

My life seemed to be a constant struggle, but I know that enjoyment should not be rare or just a fleeting state of mind. I'll make sure that enjoyment will be a constant and that struggle should be present only to overcome potential obstacles. I'll overcome the emotional issues that have been holding me back for years. I don't need to prove anything to anyone. I need to live my life for myself and Peter.

I had no idea that I had the ability to create a life I could fully love, a life that I could feel secure in while just being myself, despite all the burdens. I lived in fear of failing to live up to the expectations of others, that all I was working for could be taken away from me in an instant by a quirk of fate. The debilitating belief that I was flawed led me to allow unwelcome, constant self-doubt. As a result, I learned to live a version of life that was supposed to satisfy others, but not always myself. I learned a distorted version of living that comes from conforming to outer standards rather than from being true to myself.

In order to survive as a single mother, I've made lots of sacrifices. I regret none of them. I regret the moments when I was trying to satisfy others, people that mean nothing to me. I didn't always succeed, but I sure tried. Not anymore. Now I'm free from this burden. I don't care that I may always be marginalized by society just for being different.

I had no clear idea where my life was going. I do now. I don't live to survive anymore, but I live for the sake of living and enjoying every moment for me, for my son.

And so I look at my life now, and I relive bits and pieces of all the good things that took place. I had to face the truth of the past so that I could move forward. I have endured these last years, lost in the shadows of my past traumas.

I can see the light. Bigger than the one at the end of the tunnel. Brighter than the sun. More promising than the first flower of spring.

Now I'm ready. Ready to face the sun, to embrace its rays of light. Ready to live. Ready to be the best mom for my son. Ready to follow my passions, my dreams. I look forward to everything that is ahead of me, of us.

I see now the beauty of life.

"Life is beautiful" is what Nico would say, and you know what? She is definitely right.

# Afterword
# Life Is Beautiful

I believe that the role of every experience we have is to teach us something. If this is true, then I'm grateful for everything that happened in my life that made it possible for the three of us to meet. Maybe all the negative events prior to our meeting were representing the catalyst for some of my most important lessons and opportunities for growth.

My friends helped me see lots of things differently. They are distinct from anyone I knew.

Their presence in my life seemed necessary despite the occasional unpleasant situations. In time, I have changed. I know I would have changed even without meeting them. But due to them, I believe that I've achieved a better version of myself.

My mini-vacations and longer stays at the seaside were colorful because of them. They were something I really needed, and on top of that, I have gained so much experience.

The closeness of the sea, the fresh air, the beautiful nature wouldn't feel the same without their company.

I had no fixed obligations, except for following my passion, living my dream, and learning and getting to know them, like really know them. And because of doing that, I know now two wonderful people.

In their company or alone, I felt free to do what I wanted, when I wanted. Isn't that normal for a true friendship?

The moments of silence while spending time with them were something new to me. I was with my own thoughts but not alone. I felt these were moments of bigger self-change. A change that wasn't related to my friends. A change that was only me.

You may ask what is so special. The answer: everything.

What happened during the past few years has changed my life tremendously. One of the things that added a new dimension to it was the presence of my two best friends. Looking in retrospect, I think we were meant to meet, at precisely that moment in time. We all played important roles and had a beneficial impact on each other's lives.

ADHD is only the X-factor that makes them so special.

\*\*\*

"Life is beautiful." This is something I've often said over the years.

"Oh, not again," my little friend would say when he heard me and then he'd start laughing. He would enjoy his mocking each time he'd have the chance. He knows very well which situations would make me say the words and he would just wait for me to put them out so he could play his game.

"Life is beautiful," he surprised me recently with a big grin on his face. I looked at him surprised. This was not something I was used to. It wasn't a joke, he was being honest.

"Yes it is," I answered and smiled. A smile that seemed to have been permanently painted on my face.

He was content.
Happy.
The happiest.

# Other Titles by This Author

# LESSONS IN LIFE

## Achieving a Better "You" Through Self-Reflection

Life teaches us lessons continuously. Do we pay attention and acknowledge what we learn? Do we strive to improve ourselves, and, due to these improvements, are our lives and relationships positive influences for everyone around us?

Do you want to change your life, but you don't know where to begin? Are you in an unhappy relationship? Do you feel lonely? Can you imagine what your life would be like if you discovered what makes you feel truly alive? Are you stuck in a job you don't love? What's stopping you from taking hold of the life that you dream of?

Life's a roller-coaster. Let's transform it into genuine fun, by finding and offering only the good within us. As odd as it sounds, it takes some effort to become a good person. It demands self-awareness. It requires perseverance. You must keep an open mind about things and develop an acceptance of everything that is different, even if you don't fully understand it. However, at times, it requires nothing more than just an honest smile.

Be good! Do good! Smile! Discover a better version of yourself! Take charge now!

# MAGNETIC REVERIE

*One Woman's Struggle Between her Dreams and the Reality of Love after Newly Discovering her Sexuality*

**Lana** lives a perfect life in Washington, D.C., with her husband, Greg. Right in the middle of a peaceful and simple life, she awakens from a dream that reveals to her a new reality that questions the very essence of who she is.

Enter **Claire**, a beautiful young woman who Lana is supposedly in a relationship with.

Meandering between Slovenia while sleeping and Washington, D.C., while awake, this love story makes Lana evolve and grow.

But a decision must be made. Love wins in the end, undoubtedly, but love for whom?

**Magnetic Reverie** is the first book from **The Reverie** series.

# REVERIE GIRL

*The Sensual Journey of a Young Woman Falling Madly in Love with the Girl of Her Dreams*

**Claire** is a young woman who only accepted her sexuality after an enlightening trip to India. Soon after, she falls head over heels in love with a gorgeous girl, Lana, a woman she meets only by pure chance during a captivating encounter at Vienna's Airport terminal between flights. This love seems far from being reciprocated and rather hopeless. Or is it?

**Lana** meets Claire whilst going from Slovenia en route to America while making plans for her perfect married life. This encounter reveals the essence of who she is within. She discovers a new side to herself. She becomes torn between two worlds and must decide. Whatever her decision, there will be consequences. She can suppress her feelings and memories during the day. But can she control them in her dreams?

Will her dreams be strong enough to make Lana follow her heart?

**Reverie Girl** is the second book from **The Reverie** series.

# About the Author

**Nico J. Genes** has traveled and worked with many interesting and unique people of different nationalities, religions, and sexual orientations, all of whom helped her to understand diversity and to accept everyone just as they are.

With her first two novels, **Magnetic Reverie** and **Reverie Girl**, she broke the ice into writing successfully. From her readers' feedback and reviews, Nico can proudly say she has a solid confirmation of her skills as an established writer. An important element of her writing is that she always has a message that she wants to transmit. This can be summed up by her motto: We are all different, and that's okay!

Besides novel-writing, Nico also runs a blog in which she talks about life's issues, and gives the kind of friendly advice that everyone needs at certain points of their life. The positive feedback of her readers became her inspiration for her third book, **Lessons in Life**. Continuing her mission of welcoming all diversity and pleading for tolerance and acceptance, she wrote the novel **ADHD: Life Is Beautiful**, based on a true story.

**Nico** is eager to hear from you on www.nicojgenes.com or her social media (Facebook, Twitter, Instagram, LinkedIn, and Goodreads).

\*\*\*

Did you enjoy reading the book? You are warmly invited to leave a review on Amazon and Goodreads.
Even one sentence is greatly appreciated.
Thank you!

Ingram Content Group UK Ltd.
Milton Keynes UK
UKHW040919070323
418129UK00005B/637

9 781093 629477